Embracing Age

Global Perspectives on Aging

Series editor, Sarah Lamb

This series publishes books that will deepen and expand our understanding of age, aging, ageism, and late life in the United States and beyond. The series focuses on anthropology while being open to ethnographically vivid and theoretically rich scholarship in related fields, including sociology, religion, cultural studies, social medicine, medical humanities, gender and sexuality studies, human development, critical and cultural gerontology, and age studies. Books will be aimed at students, scholars, and occasionally the general public.

Jason Danely, *Aging and Loss: Mourning and Maturity in Contemporary Japan*
Parin Dossa and Cati Coe, eds., *Transnational Aging and Reconfigurations of Kin Work*
Sarah Lamb, ed., *Successful Aging as a Contemporary Obsession: Global Perspectives*
Margaret Morganroth Gullette, *Ending Ageism, or How Not to Shoot Old People*
Ellyn Lem, *Gray Matters: Finding Meaning in the Stories of Later Life*
Michele Ruth Gamburd, *Linked Lives: Elder Care, Migration, and Kinship in Sri Lanka*
Yohko Tsuji, *Through Japanese Eyes: Thirty Years of Studying Aging in America*
Jessica C. Robbins, *Aging Nationally in Contemporary Poland: Memory, Kinship, and Personhood*
Rose K. Keimig, *Growing Old in a New China: Transitions in Elder Care*
Anna I. Corwin, *Embracing Age: How Catholic Nuns Became Models of Aging Well*

Embracing Age

• •

How Catholic Nuns Became Models of Aging Well

ANNA I. CORWIN

Rutgers University Press

New Brunswick, Camden, and Newark, New Jersey, and London

Library of Congress Cataloging-in-Publication Data

Names: Corwin, Anna I., author.
Title: Embracing age : how Catholic Nuns became models of aging well / Anna
    I. Corwin.
Description: New Brunswick : Rutgers University Press, [2021] | Series:
    Global perspectives on aging | Includes bibliographical references and index.
Identifiers: LCCN 2020045576 | ISBN 9781978822276 (paperback) |
    ISBN 9781978822283 (hardcover) | ISBN 9781978822290 (epub) |
    ISBN 9781978822313 (pdf)
Subjects: LCSH: Aging—Religious aspects—Catholic Church. | Monastic and
    religious life of women—United States. | School Sisters of Notre Dame. |
    Aging—United States. | Nuns—Religious life.
Classification: LCC BV4580 .C585 2021 | DDC 271/.97—dc23
LC record available at https://lccn.loc.gov/2020045576

A British Cataloging-in-Publication record for this book is available from the British Library.

www.rutgersuniversitypress.org

Manufactured in the United States of America

For my grandmothers

Contents

Illustrations

Figures

Tables

Embracing Age

Introduction

One morning I witnessed my daughter noticing the signs of her body aging, growing taller; suddenly able to spit her toothpaste into the sink without the stool under her bare feet, she erupted into peals of joy, hollering, "Look! Look! I'm older!" For my young daughter, aging is a thrill, filled with new cultural practices and opportunities. She has learned the cultural script of a life course in the United States: babies become toddlers, toddlers grow into children who become old enough to go to school, to become teenagers, then young adults, and so on. Each transition is marked by new cultural expectations and practices. Like most children, my daughter is eager to embrace the signs of aging that allow her to move through these stages.

Last year, I sat on the edge of the bed and watched my ninety-eight-year-old grandmother's gaze rest on her hands, her knuckles enlarged from rheumatoid arthritis. Although I knew their curves and knobs caused her pain and embarrassed her, I always loved her hands, which she kept meticulously manicured, elegant, even as they changed shape and color over the decades. They were no longer the delicate slender fingers she had once possessed. She covered one hand with the other and remarked, "Can you believe I'm ninety-eight?" She seemed confounded by her age, not sure what it was supposed to feel like, not sure how to make sense of being old. Her rhetorical question speaks to the mysterious experience of how the passing of time translates into the experience of aging; it also reveals something about mainstream American culture. After she raised her children, concluded her career, and retired at eighty (nearly two decades earlier), there were few clear cultural practices for my grandmother to look to to make sense of this stage of her life. Her question pointed to another question: What does it mean to be old?

1

Even at nearly one hundred years of age, my grandmother was a mensch. Always perfectly coiffed, with short feathered hair and sharp glasses perched on the bridge of her nose, she always wore a collared shirt, crisply starched, under a cashmere sweater rolled up past her wrists. She possessed an unparalleled grace and composure. Although her ability to walk became limited, she continued to read voraciously, consuming the *New York Times* front to back each day. When we visited her, she would engage my two children in play from her bed, animating tiny cars, rolling them over her quilt while the children giggled. She was an aggressive competitor when they would compete to find Waldo in the popular book *Where's Waldo?* But growing older was not easy. As her ability to walk and physically navigate the world waned, her social networks constricted. She vehemently rejected friends' invitations to leave her home and move into a retirement community; she adored her home and was determined to live there until her last days. But, as is typical in American families, her children and grandchildren lived in homes of their own; many of us were a plane trip away. Living at home meant that my grandmother lived an increasingly isolated life. The majority of her friends had died, and the few who were alive could not visit her any more readily than she could visit them. She was profoundly privileged to have the assets to have in-home care from an amazing caregiver, but most of her days were spent alone with a woman who, as much as she may have felt like family to all of us, was paid to be there. My grandmother's situation was a best-case scenario: she was healthy overall; her memory was sound until her last few weeks; she had loving family members who called and visited as frequently as we could; and she had enough money to continue to live at home. But she was also startlingly alone. Despite calls and holiday visits, days, weeks, and occasionally months could go by when she saw no one but the woman she paid to live with her.

The values that my grandmother held dear were the same ones that rendered her relatively isolated. She valued her independence and control over herself and her space. These are values that resonate with many Americans. Being independent, being in charge of her home, her food, what she wore, where she went, and being able to work until age eighty: all of these were things that my grandmother valued. To give them up—to live in a community, outside her home, would mean that she would have to give up her independence and total control over her surroundings. And yet, as my ninety-eight-year-old grandmother grew older, her children and grandchildren wondered how long she would be able to live in her home and how unbearable it would be if she had to be forced—by an illness, ailing body, or depletion of funds—to move out of her home. These were very difficult conversations for my family to have. Speaking about what would happen if my grandmother declined, or speaking about the decline we noticed unfolding, felt like an affront to her person. When family members noted aloud that she was declining, that her memory and body were fading, these conversations were usually held quietly, outside of my grandmother's earshot; we struggled to know how to talk to each other and to my grandmother about her aging process. As Americans, we did not have practice speaking about it with even a shadow of the assurance or clarity I have when I speak to my daughter about her own aging process.

Aging and decline are topics American cultural norms teach us to avoid. When the topic of aging comes up in American conversation, it is often in the context of extolling a person's skill at avoiding aging: "You look so good!" "She's so active and healthy!" "You don't look a day over 60!" When discussions of aging do come up, they are often framed as if they are a problem: "Oh dear, she's losing her memory," or "He's not as active as he once was." Outside of the stream of advice on how to avoid aging, or at least avoid the appearance of aging, American society offers paltry few examples of how to grow older. While my daughter has a wealth of cultural models for her stage of the life course, with a robust community of other children, parents, and grandparents to help scaffold her aging experiences as she goes from six to seven, and from twelve to thirteen, and eventually grows into an adult, my grandmother has no parallel models. There were no cultural practices for her to look to as she entered older age. When my daughter is a preteen, gazing into a future when she might be a teenager, American culture will offer up models for her to consider and compare herself to. Her friends will have quinceañeras and b'nai mitzveh; she will see some teenagers rebelling and others sailing smoothly into young adulthood. There will be books and TV shows that portray adolescents moving through the world.

On our last visit, my grandmother looked significantly different than she had six months earlier. Her body sank slightly lower into her pillows and she had an oxygen tube in her nose. While my son ran right up to her bedside and leaned over to give her a hug, my daughter hung back and clung to me, her body stiff against the sight of her great-grandmother. When I moved forward to give my grandmother a hug, my daughter started to cry. She was terrified. In mainstream American culture, as in many postindustrial cultural spaces, children and older adults are segregated from each other in everyday life. Even though my daughter encounters babies and children, teenagers and adults, American children like her rarely inhabit intergenerational spaces in which older adults in their eighties or nineties meaningfully interact with children or young adults.

The most prevalent cultural models of aging we encounter in the United States are idealized models of individuals maintaining a process of "ageless" aging, an unchanging adulthood marked only by a passing of time. This cultural ideal, that model of individuals growing older in years without appearing to age at all, is one that permeates American culture (Applewhite 2016; Lamb 2014). Despite these ideals, in lived reality humans do not grow older in years without visibly aging. In addition to the visible evidence of aging, such as wrinkles, in the United States, 80 percent of older adults experience one chronic disease and 68 percent of older adults are living with at least two chronic diseases (National Council on Aging n.d.).

This book examines a community of individuals whose experiences of aging profoundly contrast with mainstream American aging trajectories. Epidemiologists have found that American Catholic nuns experience longevity and remarkable health and well-being at the end of life. They also live in cultural communities that provide a model for how to grow old, decline, and die that is both embedded in American culture and quite distinct from other American models, such as the one my grandmother experienced. In mainstream American society, my grandmother grew older in a cultural context in which aging is seen as a "problem," a state to be avoided as long as possible, a stage that threatened her ability to exert values that remained dear to her—independence, autonomy, and control over her surroundings. Aging in American Catholic convents is significantly different. Catholic nuns do not just age more "successfully" than their lay peers; most also practice a culture of acceptance and grace around aging. In many American convents, aging is a natural part of the life course, not something to be feared or avoided. Examining the culture of aging in an American Catholic convent reveals that human aging is not simply a biological process, a ticking on of years and the wrinkling of skin. The physical experience of aging is shaped by how we understand the process. The cultural context in which we are embedded shapes each of our aging trajectories. By examining Catholic nuns, a group that has been documented to age with grace and positive health outcomes, we see how specific cultural practices shape the process of growing older. A close look at their lives will reveal the connections across culture, language, and the experience of aging.

Aging in American Convents

American Catholic nuns experience greater positive physical and psychological health outcomes than their peers. As a whole, they have been documented to experience not only longer lives but also greater physical health and psychological well-being as they age. There are a number of straightforward factors that contribute to the nuns' health, such as consistent nutrition and higher education, but the story of their remarkable health and well-being in older age is not as simple as higher education and nutrition. The nuns' positive health outcomes are also shaped by their cultural practices. How they pray, how they speak to each other, how they offer and receive social support, and how they understand what it means to be a human growing older in years: all of these cultural practices profoundly shape the nuns' experiences of aging, pain, and the end of life.

A launching point for my research was the work of epidemiologist and Alzheimer's disease specialist David Snowdon, who documented that

Catholic nuns experience happier and healthier lives than do their lay counterparts. Snowdon and his team conducted a longitudinal study of 678 Catholic nuns from the School Sisters of Notre Dame, finding that the nuns lived longer than their lay peers. The sisters who participated in Snowdon's study were found to have "lower all-cause mortality rates than did the general population, and this mortality advantage increased over time" (Butler and Snowdon 1996). These sisters were 27 percent more likely to live into their seventies than were their lay peers, and their likelihood of living longer increased with time.

There have been hundreds of articles published on aging among American Catholic nuns, the majority of which address the development and neurobiology of Alzheimer's disease (see, for example, Riley, Snowdon, and Markesbery 2002; and Snowdon et al. 2000). In May 2001, the cover of *Time* magazine depicted a portrait of a nun in a habit, smiling above the heading "Believe It or Not, This 91-Year-Old Nun Can Help You Beat Alzheimer's." In addition to popularizing the notion that nuns age well, this research has helped gerontologists understand some of the factors that contribute to American nuns' well-being at the end of life. For example, one study found that the more years of education nuns had received, the more cognitively robust their minds were at the end of life. Education seems to have buffered cognitive decline and reduced the risk that the nuns would express dementia in later life (Butler, Ashford, and Snowdon 1996; Mortimer, Snowdon, and Markesbery 2003; Snowdon, Ostwald, and Kane 1989). Snowdon notes that sisters with a college degree were more likely to live into old age and to "[maintain] their independence without requiring nursing services or help with self-care tasks." He adds, "Not only did the less educated sisters have higher mortality rates, but their mental and physical abilities were much more limited if they did reach old age" (2001, 40).

Another study analyzed writings and personal narratives written by the nuns when they entered the convent. It appears that lower linguistic ability early in life has a strong relationship to poor cognitive function and dementia in late life (Snowdon et al. 1996). In other words, the nuns who used more complex language in their written narratives when they were young were more likely to maintain greater cognitive function as they aged. Another linguistic analysis of the nuns' archives found that positive emotions were associated with longevity six decades after the nuns had written the narratives (Danner, Snowdon, and Friesen 2001). Whatever was captured by the words describing positive emotions in the young nuns' narratives (perhaps emotion, psychological state, an orientation toward the world, or a sense of obligation to express a particular emotional outlook, which cannot be identified without ethnographic data) predicted the length and health of the nuns' lives. The expressions of language, therefore, seemed to be powerfully correlated with health as the sisters aged.

In his 2001 book *Aging with Grace*, Snowdon suggests that faith, community, and attitude contributed to the nuns' record of healthy aging. But, as he points out, the question of how these spiritual and social practices contribute to the nuns' experiences of health and well-being could not be answered by the largely quantitative data he gathered. Snowdon suggests that the methods of his field, epidemiology, are not designed to examine how and why prayer, social support, and life in a religious community contribute to positive health outcomes. This, however, is precisely what anthropology is designed to do. Anthropologists examine the everyday practices that shape the way people live—the way they speak, the ways they interact with each other, and the ways they make meaning in the world. Linguistic anthropologists examine the way people communicate. Anthropological methods are designed to examine the institutional and personal histories, socialization, and everyday practices that shape people's experiences in the world to understand their patterns and logic. While epidemiological work with American Catholic nuns is able to demonstrate that certain factors correlate with certain health and longevity outcomes, only by examining the rich context in which the nuns live, in which they learn to be in the world and to experience their bodies as aging, can we begin to develop sophisticated hypotheses about how specific practices contribute to the story of the nuns' well-being in later life.

In my own fieldwork with nuns I have found that the way they speak, engage with the world, and think about aging matters. The prayers they repeat each day shape the ways the nuns see their bodies, as well as how they think about what it means to grow older and eventually meet death. Some elements that contribute to the nuns' well-being will not surprise the reader—for example, having a sense that one will go to heaven makes it less scary to approach death. There are other things I have found in my research that have changed how I, myself, think of aging, time, and the body. In the following chapters, I tell the story of how the interactions the nuns have with each other and with the divine help promote the physical and psychological health benefits they experience as they age. Many components of this story are only revealed through close attention to language: the nuns tell stories, make jokes, and offer blessings to meaningfully engage with their peers who have cognitive or physical impairments. Through prayer, the sisters are able to communicate key cultural values, such as how to age with grace. Prayer becomes a mode of socialization into particular attitudes and practices toward aging; it is also a way for the sisters to garner social support from each other and from God.

Most strikingly, I have observed that the nuns regularly and consistently accept the body's decline. As they become infirm, notice their memory deteriorating, or receive a cancer diagnosis, they meet these changes with a sense of acceptance. The sisters present a model of aging that radically contrasts with typical American understandings of what it means to grow older. For most Americans, aging is a problem; think, for example, of my grandmother's simple act of hiding her arthritic fingers from view. Instead of learning acceptance and grace in the face of older age, most Americans learn from our communities and institutions that older age and decline are a problem. They imagine the physical and cognitive decline that accompanies aging to be unequivocally bad. Unlike my daughter, who triumphantly anticipates each next stage in her life, most American adults expend energy trying to erase the evidence of time's passing. As confirmation of this cultural trend, in 2020 the antiaging products market in the United States was estimated to be worth $14.2 billion (Globe Newswire, 2020).[1] While the convent where I did my fieldwork is in the United States, the attitudes the nuns cultivate about aging—which they began learning the day they walked into the convent as girls, and will engage in until the day they die—are distinct from these mainstream American ideals. This tells us something about how culture works. For American Catholic nuns, it is not the larger American cultural notions of aging that primarily shape their experiences of aging. Even though these women were born into American homes, watched American television, and interacted with other Americans, it is the cultural community of the convent that shapes how they experience aging. The cultural practices most close to them in the convent reweave their understanding and experiences of aging. As we will see, this reweaving involves deep historical practices as well as contemporary practices in which the nuns actively learn and relearn what it means to grow old.

In the convent, the passage from adulthood to older adulthood is marked as normal, natural, and part of God's plan. Put simply, the nuns learn to accept and even embrace the process of growing older. The sisters I met who live in the infirmary wing of the convent are joyful and peaceful. There is a sense, even for those in physical pain, that they are just where they are meant to be.

At this point in my description, I predict that many of my readers will have one of two responses. Some may assume that the nuns accept aging because they do not experience the same pain, discomfort, or chronic conditions that the readers and their loved ones have. Others may think, "Well, they're religious. They're nuns. It's just different."

I would like to address each of these points directly. First, the nuns do experience pain and illness. What is distinct about them is not that they avoid pain or illness but that they have learned to cultivate an attitude of acceptance in response to it. And second, yes, these women are nuns, yet they are also— and most fundamentally—humans. Instead of dismissing these women as "different," I challenge my readers to see how they are also the same: human, just as you are human. This book is not the story of how a group of very different people end up experiencing aging very differently than their lay peers. This is the story of how the language these women learned when they joined the convent, the language they become fluent in as they grow older, shapes their attitudes and experiences of aging.

Let us take a moment to pause on how remarkable this is. We are accustomed to a story in which things a person puts in their body (e.g., food) or does with that body (e.g., exercise) shapes that body. But that is only part of the story; the other part, and the focus of this book, is less familiar to us because it is less material. My research presents the story of how the words we learn to speak come to shape our bodies, our experiences of pain, our aging process, our very life spans. As you read this story, I implore you to imagine how the words you speak also shape your life course. We are all embedded in culture. We all produce culture. Yet cultural practices are often invisible to us. Our own cultural practices often seem like they are simply common sense or "natural" when, in fact, cultural practices are learned and relearned every day of our lives. It is through anthropology that we begin to see what is right under our nose.

Language: The Words We Speak

The question of how language impacts one's experiences in the world is not a new one. It is a topic that linguistic anthropologists have engaged with for nearly a century, a concept that coalesced most notoriously in the 1930s when Benjamin Lee Whorf and his mentor Edward Sapir posited that the structure of the language a person spoke shaped their worldview, including cognitive processes (Whorf 1997). Whorf describes observing behavior that seeded his ideas about the connection between language and worldview when he was employed at a fire insurance company. He observed that individuals consistently behaved more carelessly around gasoline drums that were empty than they did around drums that still contained gasoline (Whorf 1956). He noted, however, that the empty drums were far more dangerous, since the vapor that remained in the drum was highly explosive. Smoking a cigarette near a drum labeled "Empty" could cause a major explosion. He concluded that the meaning of the word *empty*, which in English can imply "inert" or "null and void" (1956, 135), was shaping the way individuals understood and behaved around the drums. Whorf spent much of his career exploring the ways in which language shaped experience and cognition, a field now known as linguistic relativity, and since the 1930s there has been strong empirical and philosophical research in this field (see, for example, Lucy 1992, 1997). Ultimately, after much misinterpretation and debate, contemporary work in the field of linguistic anthropology has revealed a dynamic relationship between language and experience in which language, culture, and experience each influence each other. Elinor Ochs, a linguistic anthropologist interested in the intersections between language and experience, has argued that "ordinary enactments of language," the ways in which we speak each day, "are themselves modes of experiencing the world" (2012, 142).

In this book, I tell a story about the deep entanglements between language and experience. The words we speak do more than simply describe our experiences in the world. When we speak, we shape our experiences through the very act of communicating. It is this vision of language that will carry us through the book: we will begin to see in detail how the ways in which a group of Catholic nuns speak shapes their experiences of aging and their bodies.

From the nuns I worked with, we will learn that the "secret" to aging well is not to avoid aging but to embrace it as a normal part of the life course. This theme—embracing and being embraced—runs throughout the book. A big part of this story is the creation of a community in which the sisters embrace each other. We will see that this interdependence is not always easy; embracing each other does not mean that the sisters always *like* each other. Nevertheless, they learn to support each other as they age and as they teach each other how to age well. The sisters I worked with learn the language of acceptance and social support at the dinner table, while playing cards, while chatting in the hallways, during Mass, and—as we will see—through prayer. We will see that in the convent, prayer is about much more than speaking to a divine being; it is also a way for the nuns to communicate needs, to support each other, to ask for help, and to teach each other how to be in the world. Prayer is also a mode through which the nuns practice feeling embraced by God, sometimes quite literally picturing themselves in his arms. Together we will look at the nuns' language and their everyday cultural practices to learn just how powerful language can be. We will see how words have the power to shape our very experience of being in the world.

A Note on Terminology

While the terms *elderly*, *old*, and *senior* have become controversial, with movements pushing to replace them with less stigmatized terms, such as *older adult*, I choose to continue to use these terms for two reasons. First, as will become clear in the ethnography, the nuns themselves do not problematize the process of aging and in fact seem to embrace the process of growing old. As such, I have never understood the sisters whom I write about to have any problem with these words. As an anthropologist, I strive to use the terms that a community itself would use. Second, while some people have made the argument that one should avoid these terms in order not to stigmatize older adults, changing the terms alone will not effectively counter any stigma. If one's goal is to reduce the stigma that North Americans and others experience and produce around aging, one must do the harder work of facing the root cause of the stigma itself: the values people have around aging and the life course. The nuns embrace and support the aging process and provide a cultural model with which their peers may do so as well. As such, elderly nuns in the convent are not segregated or stigmatized. This process comes from their ability to embrace conversations about aging rather than avoid them. While I am not convinced that avoiding particular terms will eliminate or reduce stigma, I do think that the nuns' story, the one I strive to tell in this book, allows us to see a model in which aging, decline, and the end of life are embraced without negative judgment or stigma.

The Organization of the Book

This book is divided into two parts. Part I focuses on well-being and interaction in the convent. Part II widens the lens from social interaction to bring the social and historical context of the nuns' lives into clearer focus, illuminating how complex social and historical forms have shaped the nuns' everyday experiences.

Each chapter addresses the questions of care and prayer in the convent from a distinct theoretical angle, exploring historical changes that have impacted the nuns' lives and engaging narrative analysis, language socialization, and an exploration of the pragmatics of prayer. My goal is to use these distinct analytical perspectives to shed light on the question of how communicative and spiritual practices in a convent have shaped the nuns' experiences of aging and well-being.

Chapter 1 introduces the reader to the convent, providing an experiential outline of life in a monastic community. Chapter 2 begins to unpack the concept of aging well that underpins the central questions of this book. The chapter proposes that while the nuns are upheld as models of "successful aging," their lived experiences as they age and the cultural values they hold, in fact, contrast with the ideals presented in the literature on successful aging. I argue that the dominant paradigms of aging present in the United States are not only problematic but also inaccurate, and I suggest that a more accurate model of aging well should include a notion of acceptance or, as in the title of the book, embracing age.

Chapter 3 explores prayer practices in the convent to understand how prayer is used to garner social support and as a mode of *language socialization*. Socialization, sometimes called enculturation, refers to the process through which individuals learn the cultural norms and practices of their communities. The process of socialization often occurs below the level of consciousness—for example, as children learn that there are certain expectations for boys in contrast to girls or as children learn to decode what practices are polite or impolite in society. As we are communicative creatures, much of the process of socialization occurs through language. Sometimes the process is explicit, as in a reprimand: "Don't say that word. It's rude!" More often, socialization is implicit as individuals learn norms by watching others.

Elinor Ochs and Bambi Schieffelin, who coined the term *language social-ization*, find that the socialization process is dynamic: individuals are social-ized *to* language as they learn to become competent speakers with particular ideas about the languages they speak and hear, and they are socialized *through* language as they learn about their communities through language (Ochs and Schieffelin 1984; Schieffelin and Ochs 1986). While socialization is often asso-ciated with childhood, chapter 3 explores how language is used in the convent to socialize older sisters into particular attitudes and orientations toward aging. Chapter 4 focuses on the problem of communicating with individuals who have communicative impairments. The nuns regularly engage older sisters who cannot or do not speak clearly in dynamic, linguistically rich interactions. This is unusual in the United States, where elders, especially those who are commu-nicatively impaired, often experience social isolation. The chapter outlines strategies the nuns use to engage fellow sisters who cannot or do not speak clearly or at all.

Part II of the book delves into the particular social and historical patterns that together create the institutional setting the nuns live in, and its chapters look closely at the role of the Second Ecumenical Council of the Vatican, or Vatican II, in the nuns' lives. Vatican II, which came about in the 1960s, pre-sented major historical changes within the Catholic Church. As the reader will see, for the sisters who lived through that period, the institutional changes that accompanied Vatican II touched nearly every element of the sisters' lives. Together we will explore how these changes shaped the nuns' aging trajectories.

Chapter 5 uses narrative analysis to explore how prayer practices in the con-vent have changed since Vatican II, and demonstrates how habitual linguistic practices such as prayer shape both the nuns' experiences and understandings of God and their understandings and experiences of their bodies and pain as they age. Chapter 6 examines historical understandings of pain in the Catho-lic Church, exploring how the meaning of pain has changed over the past century. This change is mirrored in the nuns' lives and is evidenced in the way the nuns talk about pain as they age. The chapter suggests that dual notions of the meaning of pain present a paradox as the nuns seek to "save" the body, or heal, while also accepting bodily decline. Pain has a complex cultural history for the sisters, emerging as both a sacrament and an indication of medical need. This paradox offers insight into the historical and embodied narratives that shape the nuns' understandings of their own aging bodies. Finally, chapter 7 explores the theological notion of *kenosis*, or the emptying of the self, that underpins the three vows the nuns take: commitments to poverty, chastity, and obedience. The chapter aims to show how habituated cultural patterns shape the nuns' attunements to the world, demonstrating how the practices of emptying the self of attachments have allowed some nuns to also let go of attachment to the body as they age.

The Audience(s)

Different audiences will likely find different elements of this story intriguing. Gerontologists, specialists on aging, and policy makers, as well as individuals who are themselves older or interacting with older relatives, may be interested in learning what contributes to the nuns' well-being as they age. These groups may be interested in following the arguments in each chapter that demonstrate which elements of the nuns' lives seem to contribute to their well-being, as well my argument in chapter 2 that although the nuns experience remarkable positive health outcomes, their stories nevertheless provide a counterpoint to the popular successful aging paradigm. I will argue that the contemporary paradigm is not only problematic because it constructs decline as a moral failure but also that it is inaccurate because the very communities upheld as exemplars of successful aging, such as the nuns, do not adhere to tenets of the current paradigm. In fact, there is no evidence that the health outcomes we associate with the paradigm are tied to the cultural assumptions behind it.

Anthropologists may find my arguments about the role of habitual practice—and its link to experience—absorbing and will likely be interested in the analysis of how habituated practices come to shape the nuns' embodied attunements. As a whole, the book follows Pierre Bourdieu's practice theory (1990) by exploring how cultural systems—in this case, the religious and cultural practices within a convent—become imprinted in the body. The book examines the social structures that shape individual experiences, such as the organization of time and prayer in the convent, as well as the habitual communicative practices that dynamically shape the nuns' experiences of aging. And it attends to how practice, agency, and cultural structures interweave into the fabric that renders experience meaningful. The book aims to trace these attunements as they have been shaped over time.

Students, especially those new to anthropology, may find the methods in this book most interesting. When I teach ethnographies in my anthropology courses, I often ask my students, "What did this approach teach us that we would not have learned had the author used other methods?" If you are a student reading this, you may find it valuable to track how the methods I use reveal different elements of the nuns' experiences. You might ask, "If this topic had been studied by an economist or a theologian, how might the methods and the analysis be different?" You will find that, as a linguistic anthropologist, I pay close attention to language and to experience. Readers not accustomed to encountering long transcripts may find these new or possibly disconcerting, but it is this close attention to language that will allow us to see how social interaction shapes the nuns' lives. Similarly, the fact that I use the psychological anthropologist's tool of person-centered interviews allows me to analyze how history, culture, and religious practice intertwine in individuals' lives. These complex histories, for example, might not reveal themselves if this book had been written by a psychologist studying nuns in a lab or an epidemiologist gathering survey results and medical data.

The book as a whole provides a story of how this particular group of American Catholic nuns became models of healthy aging. Some of the chapters use the microinteractional methods of linguistic anthropology to show how prayer and social support happen in the convent where I worked. Other chapters rely more heavily on my training as a psychological anthropologist as I focus on the ways in which the nuns make sense of their world. It is this combination of linguistic and psychological anthropology that sets this book apart from other ethnographies in the field.

I hope that the reader will walk away thinking about aging and the life  course in new ways. I hope to inspire the reader to ask critical questions about the way gerontologists, other researchers who study aging, and especially popular discourses in the United States address aging. And finally, as I hope for my students, I hope that the reader who has never before picked up an ethnography will walk away from this book with an appreciation for the power of anthropology. Ethnography allows us to answer questions that no other field can answer, such as the one this book is dedicated to uncovering: How do the words we speak influence our well-being as we grow older?

Part 1

Being Well in the Convent

• •

Prayer and Care in Interaction

1

Life in the Convent

• •

In 1947, when Sister Betsy[1] was seventeen years old, she took her vows with a few dozen other girls between the ages of sixteen and nineteen. Dressed as Christ's bride in a simple white gown, she prostrated herself on the cool gray marble floor, symbolizing her death to the outside world; after this day she would no longer be the master of her own destiny. She would no longer make decisions about where to live or whom to spend time with. She would no longer be known by the name she had been given at birth, Evelyn. From now on she would use the name the Mother Superior had given her: Sister Elizabeth, or Betsy. When she took her vows she understood "a little bit about life" in the convent because she had grown up near it and been educated by the sisters who lived there. She joined because she wanted to "do something hard for God" in gratitude for all that God had done for her, adding, "I knew we couldn't go home. I gave up that, so I gave up a lot. We couldn't go home, we couldn't write all the letters we wanted to write. We couldn't eat when we wanted to, it had to be a special time or something like that. So all those things put together, made it . . . made it . . . I knew what I was getting into, and but I still wanted to do it. And, I just stressed the words, uh, *something hard for God*."

Sister Betsy grew up in what she described as a happy family. She was the middle child, with two older brothers and two younger sisters. Her family lived close enough to the Sisters of the Sacred Heart Convent that she could see its chapel steeple from her home. She told me that, as a child, when she looked at the convent she could see herself inside its red brick walls. She said, "I loved God, I just loved Him so much." She said she knew the break from her family would be hard. Her family drove her to the convent with the items she was required to bring—among them sensible shoes, socks, and a woolen habit.

As a novice in the convent, Sister Betsy rose before dawn for morning prayers and prayed scripted words at prescribed times throughout the day. She was taught that when she washed she should recite "Crucified Jesus, cleanse me from sin through thy precious blood flowing from Thy sacred wounds." When getting dressed, she recited a prayer for each piece of the habit she put on. As she tied the girdle, she recited "Jesus, my beloved spouse, unite me so closely to Thee that I may remain Thy faithful bride forever." Each word, even in her silent prayers, was proscribed by the convent authorities. As she did her chores in the kitchen and swept the halls, she was not to chat with her peers but rather to silently recite scripted prayers.

She memorized prayers, which she would learn to speak aloud throughout the day. Novices were taught that these prayers should take the place of idle thoughts or chatter. Sister Betsy's contemporary, Sister Agnes Marie, described working in the convent kitchen peeling potatoes with other young sisters. The sisters were not allowed to make conversation with each other; instead they were to repeat short prayers called ejaculations or aspirations, designed to be memorized and repeated throughout the day.

Sister Agnes Marie described a moment when she was working with other young sisters in the kitchen: "We would recite ejaculations hour after hour. We had a potato peeler, this big thing where the potatoes rolled around, but we novices after breakfast and after prayer had to eye the potatoes. We didn't chat and giggle. We eyed the potatoes with ejaculations. So, someone would begin an ejaculation, 'May Jesus have mercy on us,' and then everyone would continue that until someone else began a new one."

Eventually Sister Betsy worked and lived outside the convent, first as a grade school teacher and later as a nurse. At the end of each school year she would pack her meager belongings in a wooden trunk and return to the convent. She would sit with more than six hundred other sisters on wooden pews in the cool air of the chapel until she was handed a slip of paper with her "obedience" written on it. Only then would she know if she was to return to the rural schoolhouse where she taught grade school or if she would be sent to a new school, a different position—or, perhaps, as a missionary, she might be sent abroad.

When I met Sister Betsy she had already served nearly seven decades in the convent. At the time we met, she spent her days sitting in a plush blue recliner in her small room in the convent infirmary. She had back trouble and was in constant pain. Her sisters, the other nuns, would come to her room throughout the day to hold her hand, pray and sing hymns with her, and deliver Holy Communion. Despite the chronic pain, she was full of life. Her body was hunched and crooked and she was plagued with spinal pain that would only worsen with time, but her laughter rang with unbridled merriment as she told me, "I know God loves me. But not just because I'm a sister. He loves me because He made me; He created me. And God is love. And He's wonderful to me."

In the beginning I had no idea what it would feel like to live in a convent. I had spent much of my first year as a doctoral student at the University of California–Los Angeles trying to secure access to conduct research in a Catholic convent, and in the end it had been my Jewish grandmother's casual remark, "I know a nun," that led me to Sister Angelica and to the Franciscan Sisters of the Sacred Heart.[2] I had never before set foot in a convent.

The week before my trip, I attended Mass at the beautiful Saint Monica Catholic Church in Santa Monica, California. I was a bit anxious, convinced I would be exposed immediately as an outsider. I remember taking in the massive white marble walls and the glowing gold murals of Jesus and the saints and trying my best to rise and sit, to kneel and stand in rhythm with everyone else. When it was time for Communion, I followed the line of congregants to the edge of the altar where, one by one, parishioners received the Communion wafers. As I recognized the ritual unfolding before me, my heart started to pound. I knew that Catholics considered the Communion wafer to be a holy sacrament, the body of the Lord Jesus Christ. Having beforehand scoured all of the introduction to Catholicism literature I could find (including a black and yellow copy of *Catholicism for Dummies*), I understood that in the eyes of Catholics, to take Communion without being a baptized Catholic would be a sin. I inched closer and closer as the priest placed the Eucharist in each congregant's open palms and silently panicked. How could I avoid the impending placement of the Eucharist on my hands? How could I communicate that I am not Catholic? How could I avoid disrupting the sacred silence that filled the chapel? Why was I so stupid as to follow everyone out of the pew? Should I just run out of line? I felt naïve, panicked, and deeply out of place. Months later, at Sister Betsy's convent, I knew how to rise and sit in tempo with the nuns, how to quietly cross my arms over my chest at the altar so the priest knew to offer me a blessing instead of Communion. As the rituals became familiar to me, I would occasionally find myself quietly laughing at my first humiliating experience of Communion, grateful that my singular test run and awkward encounter occurred in Santa Monica, far from the Sisters of the Sacred Heart Convent.

✦

Arriving at the Convent

When I landed at the small Midwestern airport for my first visit in 2008, Sister Angelica, who knew my grandmother from her time in New York, met me at baggage claim. She wore blue slacks and a white blouse. I identified her by the large silver cross she had told me would be pinned to her collar. Soon I would learn that to anyone in this part of the Midwest, the silver cross with a relief of the crucified Christ signaled that the wearer was a sister in the community. Sister Angelica wrapped me in a huge hug and a warm smile. I felt relieved to have recognized her, yet still anxious about our journey to the convent.

Sister Angelica walked me to the curb, where I met a second nun. Sister Paula had taken time from her work in the convent's archives to drive Sister Angelica to the airport. They had signed out one of the convent's modest "community cars" weeks before for the event of my arrival. In a few moments I found myself, the daughter of a Jewish father and a nonpracticing Catholic mother from New England, sailing down a highway in a small car on a humid June day to a Catholic convent with two nuns I had just met. We were on our way to the motherhouse, the central convent where all of the sisters had been trained as novices and where they returned for holidays and retired after they could no longer work.

From my place in the back seat, I watched the small city recede and the countryside emerge, revealing increasingly varied shades of green as we drove to the convent. The car rose and sank over small hills, passing field after field of calf-high corn, handfuls of lazy spotted cows, and the occasional farmhouse and sundrenched red barn. The green was interrupted on occasion by a massive parking lot yawning against a big box store. I was struck by how different this part of the country was from the places I had lived (the Northeast, California, and Arizona). Many people were farmers, with roughened faces and faded jeans. Billboards on the highway advertised pro-life messages asserting "Abortion Is Murder," and waves of corn nodded across the horizon.

After an hour we turned off the two-lane highway and drove over gently sloping green hills past modest homes, family farms, and fields of corn. At the top of one hill, Sister Angelica whispered, "Look, look. Just through the tops of those trees you can see the spires of the convent church." She told me that each year at Christmas, when she returned to the motherhouse from her position teaching in New York, she would eagerly anticipate seeing the spires, the sign that she had arrived "home." As we descended into a small valley, the spires became prominent, looming like protective parents over the sleepy town.

Nestled in its small town, the convent felt removed from the bustle of the outside world. Only six hundred people, including the sisters, live in the almost entirely Catholic town.[3] Two of the town's residents are priests; one serves the convent community, and the other serves the town church, which stands only a block away.

Inside the Convent

The motherhouse and its adjoining buildings were built to house over six hundred nuns. Now, the Franciscan Sisters of the Sacred Heart number only 250. More than half of these women work outside the convent as teachers, missionaries, or administrators. The convent houses over one hundred retired nuns, ranging in age from their seventies to their nineties, along with a few centenarians, all of whom returned from their work to retire in the convent. They now live full-time in the convent, where they have access to nursing care if they need it.

The nuns are both of this place and separate from it. They have far more education than most in the surrounding community; they are more likely than their neighbors to have traveled, whether for work, on pilgrimages, or as missionaries to Native American communities, China, or Oceania. Many of the nuns are far more politically liberal than people in the surrounding community, actively supporting social causes for peace, justice, and tolerance. Both before and after retirement, many of the sisters worked with local immigrants, with migrant workers, in prisons, and with people in rural and urban areas struggling with poverty.

Most of the sisters joined the convent as sixteen- to nineteen-year-old girls. In life history interviews I conducted with thirty-one of the nuns, most of them described having a meaningful relationship with at least one sister from the Franciscan Sisters of the Sacred Heart community as they were growing up. The majority of the sisters went to Catholic school, and many told me that as adolescents they desired to emulate the sisters who had taught them.

Sister Carline's story is exemplary of many of these narratives. She told me about her admiration for a sister who taught her in elementary school:

> I was taught by one of the Sisters of Charity and I really loved her and all sisters. And even at that time, in my little mind, I wanted to be like that, I wanted to be like her. And then as time went on, I put it in the back of my head. I dated and did all the things you're supposed to do as you're growing up and going to high school, going to games and all that. Then we moved [here][4] and I had the Franciscan sisters. And I really loved them too. There was just something drawing me to them.

Ultimately, one of the Franciscan Sisters of the Sacred Heart who taught Sister Carline in high school took her to visit the convent, and by that Christmas she had decided to join.

Sister Genevieve told a similar story. When I asked her what it was about religious life that had attracted her, she replied, "I think it was that the sisters were happy. They were excellent teachers, and I liked to study and I wanted to be a teacher. And so I was attracted to that, I think, because of their example and because I wanted to be like them." The themes that emerge in the nuns' stories about why they joined the convent highlight many mainstream American cultural values. The common themes of individual choice, happiness, personal fulfillment, and life satisfaction, for example, crosscut most of the sisters' narratives. <u>Sister Genevieve said that the reasons she joined were not the same as the reasons she stayed;</u> while she joined because she wanted to emulate the happiness and joy she saw in her teachers, she stayed because of the social bonds. When I asked her to expand on that, she said, "One [reason] is the bonding you get in religious life. Religious life is a family. I love it here. But also it's a real commitment to the life. Commitment to the vows, and a commitment to just living in community."

As Franciscans, the nuns see themselves as the "heart of the Church," emphasizing Saint Francis's and Saint Clare's teachings of contemplation, peacemaking, poverty, care for the poor, and care for the earth. More than once I heard the metaphor that Jesuits are the "brain of the Church" while Franciscans are its heart. The sisters see themselves as committed to prayer, presence, and service. Saint Francis, the founder of the Franciscan order, wanted, in Sister Angelica's words, all people to "be fools for Christ; live a life of joy that results in peace." As Franciscans, the sisters strive to foster Saint Francis's doctrine of peace, joy, and love through Christ.

The sisters described a powerful sense of love and gratitude for God and what they perceived God had already given them. For example, Sister Betsy, an elderly nun confined to her room as a result of severe back pain, described feeling overwhelmingly grateful for her life. She said that she had a "happy family life" and told me that she had joined the convent because she "wanted to do something hard for God." She wanted to serve God as an expression of gratitude for what she understood herself to have received in life.

Sister Angelica echoed this notion of gratitude and giving back: "I didn't go to the convent to get something out of it. I wanted to give something *to* it. I wanted to work for God; I fell in love with working for God and his people. What a wonderful thing, to help people see value in loving and knowing God."

When they joined the convent, most of the nuns understood that life there would be hard work. Most of them grew up in big families with many siblings and spent the hours before and after school working on their family farms, raising their younger siblings, and helping their mothers with housework. In these large Catholic families with four to fifteen children, it was expected that one or two of the children would join the Church as nuns or priests. Many of the nuns had brothers who had attended seminary, and a few had siblings in the convent with them. During my first few months at the convent, I met three sisters who had joined together and were in their late nineties. I also met a pair of identical twins who had joined together decades earlier and now lived next to each other in retirement.

Most of the nuns I spoke with told me that their parents accepted their decision to join the convent and seemed proud to have raised a child who would devote herself to the Church. Many saw the process of "giving" a son or daughter to the Church as a form of devotion. Only a few of the nuns discussed the decision as difficult for their families. One of the sisters who described such a conflict with her parents had been an only child, something that was quite rare—especially in Catholic families in those days. She told me that her parents were heartbroken when she told them she wanted to become a sister, and suggested that this conflict might have arisen because she represented her parents' only opportunity to have grandchildren. Her parents tried to change her mind to prevent her from joining the convent, which she described as very difficult emotionally, but ultimately, she became a nun. In this story we can see the American cultural values of self-determination at play. As a young adult, this sister was able to determine her future independently. In the United States the cultural values of independence and self-determination were valued over her kinship obligations. The convent supported her and worked to reassure the disheartened parents that the young sister's choice was a good one.

This echoes in my life!

In the 1940s and 1950s, when most of the nuns I worked with had entered the convent, adolescent Catholic Midwestern girls from farming families were rarely able to pursue degrees beyond high school. The convent provided an unusual opportunity for women to not only join a religious community but also continue their education. Most of the sisters completed a college degree, and many were asked by the convent authorities to complete master's or doctoral degrees so that they could teach in Catholic colleges and universities. Becoming a nun in the early twentieth century was a move that afforded American Catholic women a rare, socially acceptable alternative to marriage and motherhood.

Once they joined the convent, the nuns spent the first few years as postulants and then novices living in the novitiate building, a dormitory-like structure built in the 1950s on the convent property. There they received basic religious training under the supervision of the novice mistress.

In the Catholic Church, there are two types of religious orders women can join: one is an apostolic, or "active" order in which sisters, like the Franciscan Sisters of the Sacred Heart, work serving communities outside the convent walls. Technically these women are referred to in the Church as "women religious" or "sisters," not nuns; but the sisters in this community often used the word *nun* to describe themselves, and I have followed their conventions in this book. Apostolic sisters take three vows: poverty, chastity, and obedience. Nuns in contemplative orders, such as the Poor Clares and the Carmelites, take a fourth vow, a vow of enclosure, which is a commitment to live a cloistered life, praying and working inside the walls of their convents. Both communities see themselves as serving the world, contemplative nuns through prayer and service behind the walls of the convent, and apostolic nuns like the Franciscan Sisters of the Sacred Heart through both prayer and physical service in the world. Often the work contemplative nuns do inside the convent walls, work that often serves to sustain the convent financially, also serves others. This work can include farming, authoring prayer books, or producing food items to sell, such as biscuits, cheese, or wafers for Communion. Both types of communities, apostolic and contemplative, see themselves as involved in care for and service to the world. The distinction is largely in their method—serving through physical presence or serving through cloistered prayer and work.

A convent represents an interesting contradiction, as nuns separate themselves from the world in order to serve in the world. They give up ties with family and friends in order to live in community with others and with God. As Giorgio Agamben writes in his work on Franciscan monasticism, "It can appear surprising that the monastic ideal, born as an individual and solitary flight from the world, should have given origin to a model of total communitarian life" (2013, 9). When they entered monastic convent life, the sisters symbolically "died" to the material world. They had to break ties with their families and give up the possibility of marrying, having children, or working in secular jobs. Yet as Agamben points out, this break from the world is not "an individual or solitary flight," as it might have been centuries earlier. Franciscan sisters join a community of women with whom they share their physical and spiritual lives; in fact, rather than an individual or solitary existence, the nuns must negotiate shared spaces and communal living. Their lives in the convent may require far more social interaction than their lives before entering the convent did.

As they began life in the convent community, the sisters I met learned to live with their peers under a strictly regulated institutional structure. Each hour was scheduled, and meaning was ascribed to every action, from what they wore to how they moved. This strict schedule of prayer is designed to structure the day and also provide a moral structure for the nuns. According to Agamben, their daily prayers, the Liturgy of the Hours, provides "a sanctification by means of time" (2013, 29). Agamben suggests that the "strict absoluteness" of the regulation of time in monastic communities "has perhaps never been equaled in any institution in modernity" (2013, 19). The regulation of time represents a symbolic transformation for the nuns as they learn to live in a world where each moment is ordered and, through that order, rendered sacred. This is a cultural transformation as well. Time, which is differently ordered and regulated across cultural communities, is intertwined with moral meanings (Gingrich, Ochs, and Swedlund 2002). The nuns grew up in American Catholic homes where the day was divided into symbolic portions: work versus rest, the week versus the weekend, specific mealtimes; day versus night. As in any community, the division of time provided a symbolic organization to their world at home. In the convent this process is not only more strictly regulated but is also designed with an unparalleled level of detail and intentionality. Time regulation in the convent is meant to bring God's presence into each moment in the day. The process of sanctification through a daily schedule is not only theoretical or propositional, having to do with what the nuns believe but, along with other elements of the nuns' lives, is embodied, providing an experiential incarnation of sacred unity with the divine. Like the nuns' woolen habit, the institutionally assigned clothing that imbues their bodies with moral significance as a "sacred sign" (Agamben 2013, 17), the division of time is also meant to render each moment an opportunity to be in unity with the divine.

This external regulation is designed to shape the young women as they enter spiritual life. In her work on postulants in a Mexican convent, Rebecca Lester provides a psychological analysis of the process through which women entering a convent come to reshape their sense of self through the "self-conscious systematic use of bodily practices" (2005, 47). She explains, "As the postulants become habituated to the rigorous life of the convent, their bodies come to mediate between the interior sacred space of the soul and the exterior world of physical demands and temptations" (2005, 17). Lester suggests that through regimentation in the convent, the postulants she worked with felt that they changed: "They described to me a palpable sense of transformation, a feeling of becoming someone new, someone sacred. This did not mean, I learned, that the old self had been obliterated but rather that this self had become mobilized along a different trajectory" (2005, 19).

This process continues throughout the lives of the Franciscan Sisters I worked with. Behind the novitiate building, along the rolling green hills, there are rows and rows of silvery white headstones that grow smaller and smaller as they recede over a hill. It is in this cemetery that the nuns will eventually be buried with the sisters who have passed on to heaven before them. Once, as I proceeded with the sisters across the grassy lawns to the cemetery, one of them commented to me that she felt one could witness time passing by measuring the white rows of headstones; as each year passed, green fields blossomed into white crosses. Seeing the new rows of crosses advance across the hillside, the sister witnessed time creeping slowly before her, as if in a time-lapse scene in a movie. We might imagine that this, too, could be considered "a sanctification by means of time" (Agamben 2013, 29), albeit at a much slower pace. For as these crosses populated more and more of the hillside, representing the passing of time through the deaths of her peers, the sister saw time marked through the end of life and a final union with God. In the words of Sister Joan Chittister, a Catholic nun and prolific writer, for Catholics "life always comes out of death. The present rises from the ashes of the past" (2008, 19).

Convent History

The Franciscan Sisters of the Sacred Heart Convent was founded in the mid-nineteenth century. A local pastor, seeing a need for community services, established a convent to serve his small Midwestern farming community. He wrote to a Franciscan community in western Europe, and a brave nun answered his call, moving across the world to a small log cabin in the Midwest to found a religious community. The goal was to develop a convent of nuns who could provide schooling for local children and services for orphans who had survived a recent cholera outbreak. The first generation of nuns, a handful of hardworking women, expanded the log cabin into a stone building, established schools in the area, and ministered to local children. The town grew, and in subsequent decades the convent population expanded as well. The nuns established schools and extended their work to cities and towns throughout the Midwest.

In the 1960s, when many of the nuns who participated in my research were novices or young nuns, institutional change in the Catholic Church transformed their lives. The Second Ecumenical Council of the Vatican, or Vatican II, set in motion changes that radically altered the lives of Catholic nuns around the world. These changes, which included the elimination of the habit, the restructuring of institutional rules, and a democratization of convent leadership, transformed the sisters' lives. For the first one hundred years of the convent's history, from the mid-nineteenth century until the mid-twentieth, the sisters' lives had been relatively unchanged. They lived according to a set schedule, prayed the same words, and wore heavy woolen habits.

It is perhaps impossible to overstate how much of the nuns' lives and everyday practices changed during the massive social and historical shift that followed Vatican II. The nuns in the Franciscan Sisters of the Sacred Heart Community who were found to experience positive health outcomes as they aged had lived through this transformation. They grew up in a Vatican I Church and learned to be nuns in a Vatican I convent. They were socialized into a particular set of cultural practices and then took up a radically different set of cultural practices following Vatican II. During their lives, everything from the structure of the convent to the language of prayer was transformed. When we look at these sisters who have come to represent "successful aging" in the United States, and who report remarkable physical and psychological well-being, we are looking at a group of women at a very specific moment in time. To understand why these nuns experienced such well-being requires an examination of the sociohistorical circumstances that shaped their habitual practices before, during, and after this transition. As such, Vatican II plays a significant role in the story of these nuns' lives. We will return to it throughout the book.

The Twenty-First Century Franciscan Convent

When I arrived at the convent that day in June, the densely humid summer air was thick with the hum of insects and the smell of flowers and freshly mowed grass. As I stepped inside the convent, I was greeted by the cool relief of air-conditioning and the beauty of the marble steps and freshly waxed wood floors. A sense of calm permeated the space. As the seasons changed, the air outside turned crisp and the furnaces in the convent began to hum, rendering the enormous building almost startlingly warm. In the white, cold, winter months,

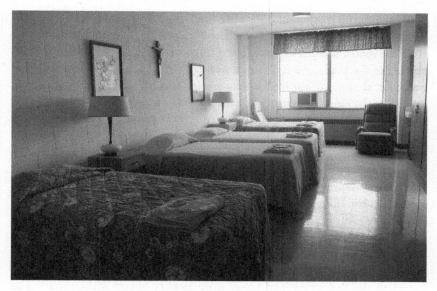

FIG. 1.1 A bedroom in the novitiate. (Photo by the author)

the heart of the convent warmed, smelling of freshly laundered hand-knit sweaters and baking bread.

The nun holding the title of congregational minister gave me permission to live in the novitiate building, which was situated across from the motherhouse facing a yard edged with flower beds. On the grounds there were spaces for prayer, benches facing grottos housing statues of Mary and Jesus, and a statue of Saint Francis, eternally feeding the birds, stood in front of the novitiate.

The novitiate was echoingly empty of novices; the building resembled a mirage of hope for a future that would never materialize. Built in the late 1960s, the two upper floors held rows of bedrooms and dormitory bathrooms with aquamarine and cream tiles and rows of showers behind pale green curtains. The expansive bedrooms (pictured in fig. 1.1) had been built as dorms with floor-to-ceiling wood-paneled closets lining the walls, built for the groups of novices meant to bunk together. The wide hallways and nearly vacant rooms spoke of a time when the community expected young women to join the convent in large numbers. When I was there, only a handful of retired nuns lived in the building, which had never welcomed the classes of novices for which it was designed.

The nuns who joined before the 1960s spoke to me of the kindness of the sisters who taught them and the opportunities behind the convent doors. The futures they described themselves leaving would have held marriages and motherhood. Entering the convent, the young sisters traded the excitement of familial love and motherhood for a lifetime in a community dedicated to education, prayer, and hard work as teachers or nurses serving those in need.

In the 1960s, as American women began to have more opportunities to work outside of the home, the number of women joining Catholic convents, especially liberal communities like the Franciscan Sisters of the Sacred Heart, began to decline. In 2012, 80 percent of convents in the United States reported that they had no new novices and 14 percent reported that they had only one (Gautier and Saunders 2013, 6). Researchers at the Center for Applied Research in the Apostolate at Georgetown University found that the number of women religious or apostolic sisters had fallen from 181,421 in 1966 to 49,883 in 2014 (Berrelleza, Gautier, and Gray 2014, 2). The Catholic Church has no official conclusion regarding why numbers have dwindled so dramatically, but the theory held by many of the sisters I spoke with was that there were now a number of opportunities through which Catholic women could gain higher education and participate in missionary or service work without joining a convent. They imagined that young women who felt the call to serve God could choose to volunteer in the Peace Corps or travel as missionary nurses without having to join a convent. The novices who did join the convent were much older than those who joined before Vatican II. As of 2012, the average age of women joining convents in the United States was thirty-nine (Gautier and Saunders 2013, 2), much older than the sixteen- to eighteen-year-old girls who joined in the first half of the twentieth century. In 2009, a National Religious Vocations Conference study found that that 91 percent of women religious, or apostolic sisters, were age sixty or older. Only 1 percent of apostolic sisters in the United States were under 40 years old (Bendyna and Gautier 2009, 27).

Sanctification through Presence

After a few days in the convent, I began to feel the rhythm of the place. In the summers my sleep would yield to the sounds of chattering birds and the quarter-hourly morning bells. I came to anticipate the voices of two sisters who passed under my window each morning before 5:30 a.m. As I showered and prepared for each day, I became aware of the quiet stirrings of a handful of retired sisters in their rooms in the novitiate as they awoke and sat in prayer. A few emerged to make tea at the shared kitchenette down the hall. Doors quietly opened and shut. The mornings were a time reserved for private prayer. Some of the nuns prayed in writing, using a daily prayer journal. Some read Franciscan prayer books. A few greeted the divine in the garden, walking the flower beds and fields, allowing the divine to emerge to them through the blades of grass and the wind. Most sat in their rooms in silent prayer.

At 6:30 a.m. many of the nuns would descend from their rooms and gather in the chapel. The slow cadence of metal walkers scraping the oak hall floors

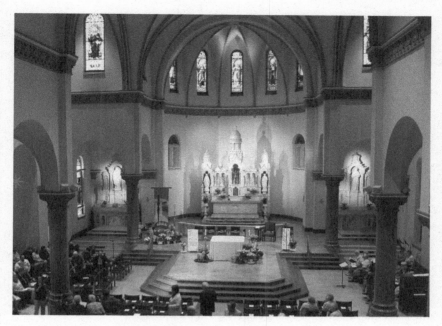

FIG. 1.2 The convent chapel. (Photo by the author)

that led to the chapel signaled to me that it was gathering time. One could judge how late it was by the tempo of shoes and tapping canes; the pace of movement quickened as the time of the Mass approached, then fell to a hush as Mass began. In the minutes before this, the chapel echoed with the soft scrub of sensible shoes on the marble floor, the creaking of wooden pews, and the rustling of clothes as the sisters crossed the center of the chapel, bowed toward the altar, and paused to dip their fingertips into the font of holy water and cross themselves. A video camera would click on as one of the retired sisters adjusted the closed-circuit video image so that the nuns who could not walk the short distance to the chapel could participate in prayer with the community. At 6:40 a.m. one of the sister's voices would break the chapel's silence as the nuns began morning prayers. Just before 7:00 the priest would emerge in the hallway and the sound of shoes moving toward the chapel increased again as the church filled with those who had made their morning prayers alone. Figure 1.2 depicts the chapel just before Mass.

After Mass, as the nuns flowed out of the stained-glass chapel doors into the hallway to the dining room for breakfast, the hush of prayer would balloon into warm chatter, hugs, greetings, and gentle embraces. Later some would return to the chapel for evening prayer, mirroring the morning ritual. Others would gather in small groups of four to eight in rooms throughout the convent with evening prayer books open on their laps. In the time between prayer time and

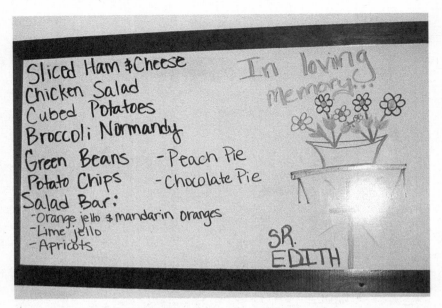

Sliced Ham & Cheese
Chicken Salad
Cubed Potatoes
Broccoli Normandy
Green Beans   - Peach Pie
Potato Chips   - Chocolate Pie
Salad Bar:
  -Orange jello & mandarin oranges
  -Lime jello
  -Apricots

In loving memory...

SR. EDITH

FIG. 1.3 A whiteboard in the dining hall. (Photo by the author)

mealtime the nuns would work or, if they could not, would pray or visit their elderly peers.

When sisters returned to the motherhouse for retirement, they often took up small duties in the convent, such as monitoring the front door for visitors or answering the phone. I witnessed sisters collaborating to find a job for a newly retired sister who seemed emotionally down or aimless upon returning. For example, one recently retired sister was asked if she could help accompany sisters to doctors' appointments; another was asked to help sort the mail. More than once I overheard sisters collaborating to find a need in the convent community so that they could ask a newly retired sister to help with it. They knew that having a way to be of service in the convent would provide meaning and structure for their newly retired sisters.

Meals were served in a large dining room in the heart of the main building. Until the last decade or so, the nuns had staffed the kitchen themselves, doing the cooking, cleaning, baking, and planning. By the time I arrived in 2008, only a few nuns worked in the kitchen and local women were employed in a number of staff positions. Before each meal, the sisters queued up in the hallway outside the industrial kitchen. Meals were served in a cafeteria-style buffet. At the entrance to the food line there was a whiteboard (shown in fig. 1.3) listing the menu and, often, decorated with a quote, a drawing, or an encouragement of some sort.

The nuns would collect their trays, silverware, and napkins and serve themselves fried chicken, barley soup, or beef brisket, with potatoes, corn, and steamed vegetables. The salad bar often had lettuce, tomatoes, and Jell-O salad. Dessert was pie, puddings, or cookies and fruit.

During the meals the nuns were warm, almost boisterous. In my first few weeks at the convent, I was taken aback by the sociality. I eventually learned that for the sisters, God existed in the chatter of the cafeteria as much as in the hush of the chapel. A few months into my time at the convent, a group of sisters told me the story of Saint Francis, founder of the Franciscans, and Juniper, one of Saint Francis's original followers. In the story, Saint Francis had suggested he and Juniper give a sermon. They went into town and casually, kindly, greeted people and spoke with them, then headed back home. Juniper said to Francis, "Holy Father, I thought we were going to give a sermon," and Saint Francis answered, "We did." The nuns followed Saint Francis's model, understanding that every interaction—even socializing over lunch or walking through town— was as sacred as any other. Speaking to a friend over lunch was understood to be as profound an expression of devotion as prayer. To build on Agamben's argument that a convent's strict schedule represents a sanctification by means of time, the nuns' post–Vatican II attitude toward sociality, which was no longer strictly regulated, could be seen as a *sanctification by means of presence.* Every action or interaction was intended to be infused with the model they saw in Christ and Saint Francis. To interact with goodwill, kindness, and generosity was to sanctify each interaction with divine love. Part of this process of sanctification through presence involved putting aside one's own desires in order to be fully present to another human. We will explore this process in chapter 7.

The lively sociality I experienced in the cafeteria, where the sisters saw themselves following Saint Francis as they cultivated the presence of God through generous interaction with others, contrasts with the ritual silence seen in many contemplative communities—such as those Paula Pryce (2019) studies in her work in the United States—where silence is seen as an agent of transformation. For the Franciscan sisters I lived with, it was through the difficult work of putting aside the ego or self while being present with others that allowed them to sanctify social interaction, to cultivate God's presence through social interaction.

The nuns strived to follow Saint Francis's model of spirituality by embodying compassion, kindness, and love while remaining highly engaged in the social world. In a lecture in the convent about Saint Clare (one of Saint Francis's first followers and the founder of her own monastic order), one of the nuns, echoing a famous quote by Saint Teresa of Avila, reminded her peers, "Jesus has no hands, no arms, no legs, so we must be his arms and legs and do his work. We must dress and act in ways that allow people to see Jesus." Humble engagement in the world was one way to do God's work: to emphasize compassion, peace, and goodness.

The Infirmary

The infirmary wing of the convent had been renovated to resemble a medical institution. It was open to the rest of the convent so that one could walk directly from the motherhouse up steps holding a polished wood banister adorned with inlaid flowers into the three-story wing. An elevator, large enough to hold a wheeled bed, was installed to provide additional access to the infirmary floors. Each floor had a nurse's station and an industrial medical bathroom with a trough-like tub equipped for bathing sisters who could no longer move their bodies in and out of a bath or shower. Across from the nurses' station was a brightly lit dining room with windows overlooking the lush convent grounds. Here the sisters who could still feed themselves gathered for midday and evening meals.

Although the convent infirmary looked medically sterile, with plastic-treated tablecloths, pitchers of water, and nurses in scrubs, it was immediately clear to me that this was no hospital infirmary. There were some lingering smells of latex gloves, cleaning solutions, and bodily fluids, but more noticeable were smells of life: the warmth of beef stew still lingering from dinner and the smells of quilts, books, and flowers.

Each door opened to a small room that held a twin hospital bed, a chair, and a TV on a bookshelf. Some of the sisters sat in armchairs, watching television. Others were reading or napping. Some were in bed. A few waved. One sister, stiff on her bed, moaned and moaned. A few, in wheelchairs, stared blankly out the window.

As I met the nuns, the contrast with other medical facilities I had seen became heightened. Sister Betsy, whom we encountered at the beginning of this chapter, was one of the first people I met in the infirmary. She spent most of her time sitting, slumped a bit to one side, her soft body spilling over the chair because her back no longer held her upright. Her room was next to the elevator. Her days were punctuated by the ding of the elevator announcing itself on one side of her and her neighbor, Sister Esther, moaning on the other side. When one of the nuns, Sister Mary, tapped on Sister Betsy's door to introduce me, Sister Betsy struggled to turn her body toward us in her chair. One shoulder sagged much lower than the other and the pale flesh on her forearm gathered on the chair where her arm rested. As we walked into her room, Sister Betsy's face lit up; she met us with a gleaming smile and warm blue eyes. Sister Mary bent down, grasping the arm of the chair to steady herself and wrapped her arms around Sister Betsy. She introduced me, saying, "this is Anna, our visitor." Before even asking why I was there or allowing me to explain myself, Sister

Betsy grabbed my hand in her warm palms and enveloped me in her smile. "Welcome, welcome!" she said, gesturing to me to pull up the one extra chair in the room and sit down.

The only similarities between this infirmary and other medical institutions I had seen were physical, not social or interactional. The patterns of interaction were distinct from what I had observed in other nursing homes and assisted living communities. As visitors passed by rooms or entered to visit, there was no hesitation before they entered. Even the sisters' attitudes seemed distinct. There was no fear in Sister Betsy's eyes. She, like almost every person I met, did not wait for me to touch her, to advance. She held me, touched me, welcomed me with her body. Even though her body was ill—chronically so and deteriorating—her way of being in her body was confident, warm, and unashamed.

While I felt the difference in the convent infirmary immediately, it has taken me years to understand the habitual practices that created it. This book seeks to share what I have learned about why aging in the convent is unique. The following chapters begin to unpack the puzzle of not only why Catholic sisters seem to experience fewer chronic conditions as they age but also why women like Sister Betsy—who live in constant chronic pain and can no longer walk, work, or even leave their room in the infirmary—seem to experience each day with remarkable peace and joy, meeting each new person with warmth and kindness. This book is as much about the puzzle of how the nuns maintain well-being as it is about what well-being means to them, and how the culture of the convent comes to shape this process.

2

Being Is Harder
Than Doing

•••••••••••••••••••••

The Process of
Embracing Aging

The idea that one group of Americans ages "better" than another group—living longer, happier, healthier lives—is quite alluring. It might inspire us to ask why and how some people achieve such impressive health outcomes while others do not. Within the context of this book, implicit in many people's curiosity to learn more is a desire to follow in the nuns' footsteps: if the nuns experience better physical and mental health, could I as well? This chapter begins by unpacking the notion of well-being and explores what it means to the sisters that they "age well." I then turn to the concept that the academy calls "successful aging," which I critique as an antiaging model, to examine how the notion of aging well has been imagined within academia as well as in popular publications and discourses. I will suggest that the popular antiaging paradigm—that of successful aging—does not merely reflect scientific findings but promotes specific neoliberal cultural values such as independence and productivity.[1] Although Catholic nuns are heralded as models of successful aging for their record of positive health outcomes at the end of life, the cultural practices and values that they demonstrate as they age in fact *contrast* with the tenets of the popular paradigm. This chapter will unpack the assumptions embedded in the current paradigm in which "success" is based on avoidance of aging. We will then turn to my hypothesis that the nuns, who are indeed healthy and happy at the end of life, experience well-being precisely because they embrace aging as a natural part of a healthy life course. I will introduce the nuns' cultural paradigm, which I call *embracing aging*.

The desire that many people have voiced to me when I have spoken about my work—to learn about and potentially emulate those who age "well" or "successfully"—is a desire that is itself wrapped up in the antiaging paradigm that dominates American[2] discourses about aging. This chapter will examine the cultural concepts and values that are inherent in this discourse, and we will find that the nuns who age with well-being do not express a desire to age "successfully" or to avoid aging. In fact, it might be the very antiaging discourse disguised as successful aging that can hamper many people's experiences of joy, peace, and well-being as they encounter older age.

Defining Well-Being

An increasing number of studies have suggested that religious practices, including prayer, meditation, and participation in religious services, aid the mental and physical health of the practitioner, promoting physical well-being and protecting against depression (Koenig 1999; Koenig et al. 1997; Newberg 2006; Strawbridge et al. 1997). Through meditation, for example, Tibetan monks are able to neurologically train their brains to reinforce "positive feelings and well-being" (Newberg 2006, 187). Other studies have suggested that religion provides a supportive relationship with a divine being (Pevey, Jones, and Yarber 2008, 55). In an interesting confluence of the biological and social sciences, work with neuroimaging has begun to document physiological changes in the brain that correlate with the religious experiences that have been documented phenomenologically—through detailed attention to individual experience—in the social sciences for decades. In the early twentieth century, William James, the first noted proponent of psychology in the United States, compared hundreds of reports of mystical and religious experiences, finding that they shared similarities that cut across cultural, religious, and theological commitments (1982). Newer developments in neuroscience are beginning to allow scientists to correlate phenomenological accounts of religious experience with mechanistic accounts of what is occurring in the brain (see, for example, Beauregard and Paquette 2006, 2008; McNamara 2009; Newberg 2006] Newberg et al. 2010a and 2010b; and Yaden, Iwry, and Newberg 2016). The studies that use neuroimaging to map these events have received massive popular attention and are indeed impressive. Yet the new scientific ability to point to the material mechanisms in the brain where these changes are happening does not answer ethnographic, cultural, and psychological questions, such as how everyday interactions shape these experiences and how these experiences might shape cultural and physiological processes like aging.

To begin to answer these questions, we must first ask, What does *well-being* really mean? What does it mean to have a high quality of life? These two terms, *quality of life* and *well-being*, are often used as synonyms. Quality of life is most often associated with external measures such as physical health, while well-being often includes measures of both subjective and objective states.[3] Across disciplines, well-being is defined as a collection of specific attributes. In psychology, for example, well-being usually refers to subjective states, including life satisfaction; positive affect, such as high self-esteem; and limited negative affect, such as anger, anxiety, depression and fear (Diener and Chan 2011, 25; Maton 1989). The field of gerontology expands this definition to include physical, social, and mental criteria including "length of life, biological health, cognitive efficacy, social competence and productivity, personal control" (Baltes and Baltes 1993a, 5). A few gerontologists also include measures of spiritual satisfaction in their assessments of well-being.

Anthropology insists that the study of well-being must be situated in cultural and historical contexts. This means that rather than defining well-being as a specific set of fixed attributes, anthropologists understand that well-being may mean different things in different cultural communities. In the introduction to their edited volume *Pursuits of Happiness: Well-Being in Anthropological Perspective*, Gordon Mathews and Carolina Izquierdo define well-being as "an optimal state for an individual, community, society, and the world as a whole" and assert that "it is conceived of, expressed, and experienced in different ways by different individuals and within the cultural contexts of different societies." They argue that since the factors that make up well-being vary across cultural contexts, it cannot be understood to be one set of attributes; rather, it must be studied through "soft comparison" using ethnography and attending to how people understand themselves in context (Mathews and Izquierdo 2010a, 5–6). In her work with the Matsigenka of the Peruvian Amazon, Carolina Izquierdo found that although "objective" indicators of physical health were increasing among Matsigenka community members, their sense of well-being was in drastic decline, as evidenced, she writes, "by an upturn in accusations of witchcraft and a general fear of the future" as the community experienced increasing encroachment from multinational oil companies (2010, 14). To draw conclusions about well-being from exclusively physical health markers without examining the social, historical, and experiential contexts can be misleading. Izquierdo shows us that well-being must be defined and examined with attention to cultural context. Similarly, in her work in an Australian Aboriginal community, Daniela Heil (2010) demonstrates that well-being can be defined in multiple and contrasting ways. In Central West, New South Wales, Aboriginal community members define well-being as a sense of kinship and being "one of us" in community. This sense of well-being runs in contrast to the Australian government's notion of well-being as necessarily individualistic.

Ethnographic studies have also illuminated how the notion and experience of well-being can vary over time. Psychological anthropologist Thomas Weisner, whose research focuses on well-being in childhood, argues that instead of a set of attributes, well-being should be understood as engaged activity. He defines it as "engaged participation in cultural activities deemed desirable by a cultural community (e.g., kinds of play, work for the family, prayer), and the psychological experiences produced thereby (such as effectance, happiness, and trust)" (Weisner 2002, 279; see also Weisner 1998). Douglas Hollan, another psychological anthropologist, introduces the importance of temporality, the idea that the passing of time that can change one's perspective, also contributes to well-being. He argues that "one's awareness of one's own state of wellness or unwellness is a dynamic and ever-changing product of the interaction of body/brain and experience" (Hollan 2010, 212). Hollan's notion of the "self-scape" captures a dynamism of the self that, he writes, "is constantly mapping its own representations of its own past experience onto the space and time of the contemporary culturally constituted world" (Hollan 2010, 214). His work adds the notion that one's experience of well-being might change over time and is dynamically shaped by one's cultural and embodied experiences in the world.

Ethnographic work that attends to well-being has increased over the years as anthropologists have turned their analytic gaze toward an anthropology of the "good." As Joel Robbins (2013) argues, the field's move to inquire after the "good" or the "ethical" cross-culturally has come as a shift away from previous decades of attention toward human suffering and pain. As Robbins suggests, while the anthropological documentation of human suffering may have arisen through a desire for compassion and a drive to do "good" ethical work in the world, it had the unintended negative consequence of furthering the notion that those under the anthropological gaze are the "other" and are reduced to what Robbins calls the "suffering slot" (Robbins 2013, 450).

Bruce Kapferer and Marina Gold suggest that when anthropologists develop overarching theories of morality or "the good," they inadvertently manifest "a moralism underneath, a repressed or suppressed moralism despite declarations against it, that extends from the Western imperialism of the past (and its ideological roots in Western Christianity secularized into an engine of modernity or the dynamics of contemporarily)" (2018a, 12). In other words, by trying to define morality, ethics or "the good," anthropologists inadvertently promoted Western ideals. Dan Kalb warns against focusing only on what people assess as the good without examining the larger structures that shape cultural notions of morality (2018, 70). Just as Carolina Izquierdo (2010) points out, when assessing well-being, it is essential to look not only at measures of individuals' well-being but also at larger social structures, such as the oil companies' encroachment on the Matsigenka, in her example, or the ideals, education systems, and cultural values that might accompany similar neocolonial expansion. Kalb reminds us that the very notion of what is good is informed by larger social structures around the individual. When these structures are unequal, it becomes impossible to assess well-being or morality without first critically examining the power dynamics of the larger social structure.

Anthropologists see the notion of well-being as both culturally and contextually flexible, encompassing culturally relevant attributes as well as a sense of temporal and social movement and possibility. Weisner's and Hollan's work remind us that well-being is not a steady state but a fluctuating experience influenced by a continually updated sense of the body in the social world. Izquierdo, Kapferer and Gold, and Kalb each remind us that experiences of well-being and the good are shaped by larger social structures and must integrate critical analyses of power. It is not enough to accept what individuals report to be good without examining how institutional, social, and capitalist forces are shaping taken-for-granted cultural patterns.

The Nuns' Sense of Well-Being

One of the first questions I addressed in the convent was whether the nuns reported a sense of well-being similar to previous studies of American nuns. I administered a questionnaire on quality of life in the convent that asked the sisters to report on their well-being in physical, psychological, social, and spiritual domains. This questionnaire aimed to address both what are considered in psychology to be internal (psychological and spiritual) as well as externally measurable (physical health) attributes.

Using the McGill Quality of Life Questionnaire (Cohen et al. 1995, 1997; Henry et al. 2008), a survey designed to measure quality of life for those at the end of life, I found that the nuns at the Franciscan Sisters of the Sacred Heart Convent residing in the assisted living and infirmary wings of the convent reported a relatively high overall quality of life.[4] When asked to rate their overall quality of life, including physical, emotional, social, spiritual, and financial aspects over the previous two days from 0 ("very bad") to 10 ("excellent"), the majority of the nuns reported a relatively high overall quality of life at level 8 (see fig. 2.1).

When asked about psychological symptoms including depression, anxiety, sadness, and fear of the future ranging from 0 (no symptoms) to 10, the nuns responses averaged 1.68 across these four psychological categories with a standard deviation of 2.03. In comparison, using a modified version of the McGill Quality of Life Questionnaire, Melissa Henry and colleagues (2008, 720) report a much higher average, at 3.98 for the same set of symptoms with a standard deviation of 3.02.[5] This confirms that the nuns report relatively high well-being for

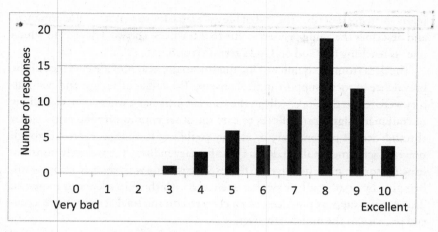

FIG. 2.1 Overall quality of life in the convent.

these psychological measures. It is worth noting that the average psychological symptoms in Henry and colleagues' report is outside the standard deviation in the convent data. The quantitative measures are useful to visualize how the nuns see themselves at a particular moment in time. This book will situate these data in ethnographic context, expanding on these quantitative measures with person-centered interviews and participant observation to establish a holistic understanding of their well-being.

The majority of the nuns in the convent understood well-being to include not only physical and mental health but—most important to them—a deep and enduring connection with the divine. The convent mission statement outlined a commitment to prayer, service, community, and connection with the divine. In my interviews with them, the majority of the nuns' definitions of well-being aligned with these values, including time and space to pray, the ability to serve those in need, and a deep connection to God.

All of the nuns, especially the older sisters, saw themselves as involved in a day-to-day process in which they strived for spiritual well-being. One of the nuns, Sister Carline, who was suffering from cancer, said that she aspired primarily for what she called "spiritual healing." She described this as "when your whole body can accept whatever is coming in your life." Sister Carline's goal, which is consistent with the model I found in the convent as a whole, exemplifies the nuns' values of serenity and acceptance of the future, which they understand to be God's path for them; I explore this model in more detail in chapter 6. Although the nuns saw God as possessing the power to intercede in the material world, they focused their prayers to the divine on requests for endurance and spiritual comfort rather than physical healing. Benedictine nun

Joan Chittister describes the end of life as "a time for surrender and acceptance" and describes the aging process as one that involves "spiritual depth" in which one "is reaching for God on God's terms" (2008, 222, 18).

The data from the quality of life questionnaire also provide evidence of the prevalence of social support in the convent. The values of service and community were realized quite vividly in the convent infirmary, where even the elderly or frail made significant efforts to care for other community members either through acts of pastoral care or, if they could not leave their rooms, through prayer. Each time I walked down the infirmary hallway I saw elderly nuns visiting those even more infirm than themselves; talking with them in their rooms; bringing by news, mail, or sweets; or sitting with them in silence or in prayer. These social support practices, often centered on spiritual activity, were a central practice in the nuns' daily lives.

Early in my time at the convent I spoke with Sister Doreen, a tiny frail sister in her late nineties who was sat in a motorized wheelchair at a small desk in her room. I had to raise my voice in order for her to hear me. I asked her how she spent her days now that she was in the convent infirmary. Without hesitation, she told me that she "visits the elderly." I am embarrassed to confess that at first, in my surprise, I did not believe her. I remember wondering who in the world could be more elderly than this tiny, frail, nearly deaf woman. The following weeks remedied my skepticism as I encountered her each afternoon, week after week, progressing down the hallways in her wheelchair, visiting the sisters who could no longer leave their rooms and praying with them or just providing company. These social support practices that Sister Doreen demonstrated were part of a vast web of social support in the convent.

When asked to rate the statement "Over the past two days, I have felt supported" from 0 ("not at all") to 10 ("completely"), nearly all of the nuns I surveyed reported feeling highly supported, with an average of 8.83 (standard deviation of 1.3); only a handful of the nuns (five out of sixty-three) reported a 7 or below (see fig. 2.2). In comparison, Henry and colleagues (2008, 720) report a mean of 7.5 (with a standard deviation of 3, indicating a wide range).

Social support has been defined as the perception that one is loved and cared for, valued, and integrated into a network of mutual assistance (Wills 1991). A more interactional approach defines social support as "the feedback provided via contact with similar and valued peers" (Gottlieb 1985, 5). Research has shown that social engagement and support from others correlates with positive health outcomes, reducing stress, and positively impacting both physical and psychological well-being (Golden et al. 2009, Golden, Conroy, and Lawlor 2009). Specifically, research has documented a connection between social

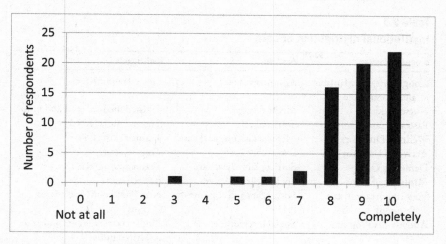

FIG. 2.2 Reported sense of support in the convent.

support and physiological and psychological function, including improved immune, cardiovascular, and neuroendocrine function and decreased depression and anxiety. Research findings have shown that social support helps buffer against the negative impacts of stress (Cohen 2004; Seeman 1996; Thoits 1995). In contrast, loneliness and isolation are linked to negative mental and physical health outcomes and higher mortality rates (Courtin and Knapp 2015; Hawkley and Cacioppo 2010).

As an institution, the convent systematically structured interactions with retired sisters in ways that afforded a tremendous amount of social interaction and care. Table 2.1 demonstrates the abundance of institutional structures designed to bring individuals into care interactions, through which the older nuns provided and received medical, social, and spiritual care.

These institutional structures put people together into situations of care, engaging a number of people at various stages of life in the work of care, including high school students from the Catholic school the sisters ran, younger sisters working outside the convent, retired nuns still living independently, and the elderly sisters (as in the prayer partners program). Table 2.1 represents structured care interactions and not the myriad of other engagements built into convent life, such as Mass, prayer meetings, recreational activities, meals, and card games. It provides a visual representation of the many structured, often mutual, care activities in the convent.

The combination of the institutional structures—programs that engage people face-to-face in various activities, along with the powerful institutional ethos of how to relate to others as one would relate to the divine—afforded a

Table 2.1
Institutional distribution of care

Group/Committee	Function	Participants
Congregational Minister and Committee	Administrative	Elected committee
Nurses/Aides	Medical care	Trained medical staff and nuns
Pastoral Care Ministers	Spiritual care	Trained nuns (RNs)
Wellness Director	Medical and physical care	Trained staff (PTs)
Activities Director	Social care	Trained staff
Dementia Care	Spiritual, medical care	Trained nuns (RNs)
Ministers of Care	Social, spiritual care	Retired nuns
Very Important Sister Program	Social care and support	Nonretired nuns and retired nuns
Adopt-a-Sis Program	Social interaction	High school students and retired nuns
Prayer Partner Program	Spiritual care	Nuns in infirmary
Regular Volunteers	All forms of care	Nuns
Individual Visits	All forms of care	Nuns, family, and friends

unique type of friendship, based on care and duty, not emotional fulfillment. As we will see in chapter 4, care in the convent was not a unidirectional activity in which one actor "provided" care to another who "received" it. Care in the convent was mutual, ongoing, and dynamic.

The quality of life questionnaire I distributed also supports the ethnographic findings that the nuns valued community and social support. When asked to rate their lives over the previous two days on a scale of 0 through 10, with 0 as "utterly meaningless and without purpose" and 10 "very purposeful and meaningful," the nuns rated their lives as highly meaningful and purposeful (see fig. 2.3). There are many components that contributed to the nuns' sense of meaningfulness. We will continue to explore these in future chapters.

While the nuns reported a relatively high quality of life in their surveys and in the ethnographic data, it is important to note that, like all humans, they also experienced vicissitudes in their emotional lives. For example, it was evident that the sisters who had returned to the convent in the previous six months seemed to experience a dip in their emotional well-being. In interviews about their years in the convent, I noticed that the sisters who had just returned often seemed glum and admitted that it had been hard to give up their lives serving the communities they had worked for. This dip in well-being was confirmed both by the head nurse and the congregational minister, who each independently suggested that this transition "home" was often hard for sisters who had spent their lives serving actively in the world. When their bodies no longer

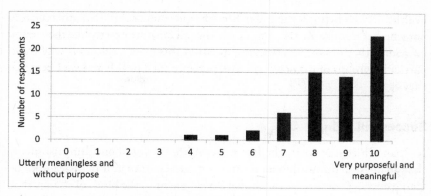

FIG. 2.3. Reported meaningfulness of life in the convent.

allowed them to be active, they had to retire to the convent. It appeared that most of the sisters adjusted in about six months to a year, at which point they seemed to complain less or not at all and to appear more cheerful and integrated in convent life. The head nurse and congregational minister corroborated this estimate as well. The quantitative data above includes sisters who had recently returned to the convent to retire, indicating that any dip associated with retirement was not significant enough to bring down the overall scores. This trend may, however, account for some of the lower scores in the survey data.

My research has confirmed that, like the nuns in School Sisters of Notre Dame, the Franciscan Sisters of the Sacred Heart seemed to experience a relatively high sense of well-being even as they aged. This well-being continued even when they could no longer work, as their bodies declined, and as they approached the final stage of life. Because of this, along with their longevity and markers of physical health at the end of life, American Catholic nuns have been heralded in the past two decades as models of "successful aging."

To be sure, it is important to note that every American nun may not be represented by these data. While the hundreds of articles Snowdon and his colleagues have published and my work with the Franciscan Sisters of the Heart provide evidence that, as a whole, these groups of women experience health and well-being as they age, one should not come to the overly broad conclusion that all nuns experience health and well-being as they age. Not only is there considerable interindividual variation in each convent, there is also variation in the cultural communities and practices across American convents. The community Snowdon worked with, the School Sisters of Notre Dame, and the community I work with are both apostolic communities in the Midwest. I chose to explore the cultural practices and experiences of well-being among the Franciscan Sisters of the Sacred Heart specifically because these women experience greater health and well-being at the end of life. The question of this book, therefore, is not whether all nuns are the same or whether all nuns are exactly like these nuns (of course they're not!). Rather, the question this book explores is why these particular groups of women seem to experience such health and well-being as they age.

Successful Aging

As Joan Chittister notes, the late stage of life "is not about diminishment, though physical diminishment is surely a natural part of it. It is, instead, about giving ourselves over to a new kind of development to the kinds of change that begin in us at the time of conception and continue in us still. The truth is we are a great deal more than our bodies, have always been more than our bodies, but it can take us most of a lifetime to learn that" (2008, 17).[6] Gerontologists and popular writers alike have enthusiastically explored why some people age more "successfully" than others and how we can all attempt to do so. On its surface, this research paradigm presents an appealing model; it is particularly attractive when compared to the models of aging it has replaced, which portrayed the end of life as a slow and steady decline. The process of growing old was once seen as an inevitable deterioration into social disengagement and physical disability (Achenbaum and Bengtson 1994; Butler 1975; Cumming and Henry 1961). Only in the past few decades have researchers who study aging ceased to describe aging as an inevitable decline into physical infirmity and social isolation. The new model that now dominates the field of aging paints a much more attractive picture: this new model that been named successful aging portrays a process in which older adults age while continuing to experience the same physical and mental health that they experienced in earlier adulthood and continue to live productive, vibrant lives. At the same time that the gerontological discourse around aging has shifted, the demographics and experience of older age has changed, as once fatal conditions have become increasingly manageable chronic illnesses through the availability of medical technologies (Buch 2015, Manderson and Smith-Morris 2010).

This new successful aging model, one that I call the antiaging model, is certainly enticing. A testament to its appeal is the proliferation of popular literature on how to age "successfully": guides to living active, productive, long lives abound. After all, what individual, steeped in a culture in which productivity and independence are the pinnacles of happiness, would not want to live a long, healthy, happy, and productive life? If the only two options are to decline into decrepitude or ski and canoe at the age of ninety until one dies peacefully in one's sleep, for most Americans the choice is obvious.

Yet exploring this paradigm reveals that this antiaging model is not so simple. I outline three central problems with the paradigm: (1) that it presents an inaccurate model of the life course; (2) that it implies that one can fail at aging; and (3) that it is a cultural, not scientific, model.

Successful Aging Presents an Inaccurate Model of the Human Life Course

The successful aging paradigm presents a model in which becoming older is merely a continuation of younger adulthood. It precludes any possibility for individuals in their older years to experience a different life stage than they did in their thirties, forties, or fifties. This antiaging model in which one does not age but simply grows older, unchanged, does not allow for older adulthood, in which obligations and kinship roles may change as individuals become the oldest generation in their families, some taking on new kinship roles as grandparents or great-aunts and great-uncles, as elders in their family or community.

In addition, this antiaging model also does not incorporate the role of death or decline, yet both are inevitable companions to life. Only rarely do people live a long life entirely free of chronic conditions and physical decline to die peacefully in their sleep in their late nineties. For most individuals lucky enough to live into their eighties, nineties, or past one hundred, chronic conditions and physical decline are an inescapable part of life, and every human will eventually meet death. While it is certainly true that particular practices such as smoking, or life events such as childhood trauma or lack of nutrition, can have lasting impacts on one's health over a lifetime, it is nevertheless a reality of being human that, if we live long enough, most of us will decline—and all of us will die. The antiaging model fails to provide an accurate account of the human life course.

Successful Aging Implies That One Can Fail at Aging

By suggesting that there is a way to age "successfully," the current paradigm necessarily implies that there are ways to age that are, by contrast, unsuccessful, that one can fail at aging. Yet no one has found a way to outsmart death. Many people who do everything "right"—eating well, exercising, and avoiding smoking and other harmful activities—also often find themselves suffering from chronic conditions such as cancer and heart disease. Furthermore, the positive health outcomes associated with the successful aging model are not equally available to all people. For instance, environmental stressors outside of people's control have been shown to have chronic negative health outcomes (Evans and Kantrowitz 2002; Gee and Payne-Sturges 2004; Kaplan et al., 2001; Marmot, Kogevinas, and Elston 1987). Poverty, racism, and social marginalization are major contributing factors to stress and illness throughout the life course. These social disparities can predict disparities in health, and illnesses linked to these disparities can in turn limit opportunities for social mobility that can impact communities for generations (Abramson 2015, 11).

A consequence to representing health in old age as "success" is that anyone who experiences illness, decreased mobility, dependence, or decline is not considered to be aging successfully. Those who experience the physical changes that often accompany aging are therefore set up to see themselves or be seen by others to be failing. Furthermore, when these fall along socioeconomic and racial lines, existing disparities are reproduced (Abramson 2015).

The term *successful aging* was first coined by Robert Havighurst in 1961 and was popularized by John Rowe and Robert Kahn in a 1997 article and 1998 book. They define successful aging as "avoidance of disease and disability, maintenance of high physical and cognitive function, and sustained engagement in social and productive activities" (1997, 439). In Rowe and Kahn's model, one's path toward older age is imagined as within an individuals' realm of control; an individual can fashion their own aging trajectory. As they note, "Our concept of success connotes more than a happy outcome; it implies achievement rather than mere good luck. . . . To succeed in something requires more than falling into it; it means having desired it, planned it, worked for it. All these factors are critical to our view of aging, which, even in this era of human genetics, we regard as largely under the control of the individual. In short, successful aging is dependent on individual choices and behaviors. It can be attained through individual choice and effort" (1998, 37).

In this description, aging is a process that an individual can control through "individual choices." This implies, of course, that if one fails to make the right choices, she might not age "well" or successfully. It also implies that if one does not age "successfully" it may be due to a failure of the individual. For people who find themselves chronically ill, living with cancer, or simply declining in old age, the burden of believing that they themselves are at fault has the potential to cause emotional distress; the paradigm itself may cause harm. The idea that one's health outcomes are dependent on individual choices is further complicated when social factors such as poverty, racism, and social marginalization—all structural factors outside of an individual's control—contribute to chronic illness.

Successful Aging Is a Cultural, Not Scientific, Model

The ideals presented by Rowe and Kahn have been taken up widely in the field of aging and gerontology and dominate popular North American conversations about aging. Yet instead of representing scientific findings, the successful aging paradigm exposes North American cultural ideals (Fabbre, 2014; Lamb 2014; Lamb, Robbins-Ruszkowski, and Corwin 2017). Sarah Lamb, who has worked with elders in both the United States and West Bengal, India, compares the conversations she has had in both places. She writes that, in India, elders conveyed an acceptance of death, saying, for example, "I say to God, 'Whenever you are ready, take me.' I am not afraid of death, because it is inevitable" and

"We have to accept decay. I have accepted." (2014, 42). She explains that in India the discourse on aging as a natural and accepted element of a good life is dramatically different from her research findings on aging in communities near Boston. In the United States, she writes, elders do not see decline as natural. Rather, they embrace the successful aging paradigm that idealizes independence and longevity. Decline and death are seen negatively, and this model promotes an antiaging message. As Lamb writes, the notion of successful aging promotes "a vision of the ideal person as not really aging at all in late life, but rather maintaining the self of one's earlier years" (Lamb 2014, 42, 45). Sociopolitical critiques have drawn attention to the ways in which the values of successful aging are intimately bound to "Western neo-liberal expectations for productivity and independence in a capitalistic society" (Fabbre 2014, 2; see also Calasanti 2004; Dillaway and Byrnes 2009; and Liang and Luo 2012).

In other words, the expectations associated with successful aging underscore Western neoliberal ideals in which an individual's value is aligned with their independence and earning power. Lamb articulates four cultural ideals promoted through the successful aging paradigm: individual agency and control, productive activity, independence, and active adulthood or permanent personhood. These ideals are set up within the literature to symbolize success, meaning that these four ideals are held up as symbols of aging "successfully." A consequence of this is that those who encounter illness, decreased mobility, dependence, or decline as they age necessarily embody the opposite of successful aging and are therefore set up to see themselves or be seen by others as failing.

While these cultural values may seem unequivocally "good" to many of my readers, they are not considered universal values across cultures. As we saw with Lamb's work in West Bengal, there are many communities that do not hold individual agency and control, independence, productivity, and permanent personhood or ageless adulthood to be necessarily good. In West Bengal, older people frequently talk of readiness for death, and "this talk of death is not limited by any means to those who are in various states of frailty but is entirely normal even among those enjoying robust physical and mental health" (Lamb 2014, 41). Acceptance and even anticipation of decline and death is seen as a normal, appropriate way to age. Just as in the United States and many places in the world it is culturally appropriate for a child like my daughter to anticipate becoming an adult and to talk about what it will be like when she is grown up, what she might do, or whether she will have children, in West Bengal it is normal and culturally appropriate for adults to anticipate decline and death as a natural, appropriate unfolding of the life course. The neoliberal values of independence and productivity are not universal indicators of a good life or a desirable way to age. They are cultural values, not human universals.

A serious problem with the successful aging model is that is that it is not scientifically accurate. Although the successful aging paradigm is promoted by scientists, including the majority of gerontologists and other scholars working at the forefront of aging research, the values promoted in the paradigm do not provide an accurate reflection of the research on individuals who experience positive health outcomes as they age. Many of the communities upheld as exemplars of successful aging—those experiencing positive health outcomes, including the American Catholic nuns we meet in this book—do not adhere to the model. The nuns uphold none of the ideological values of the successful aging paradigm. In fact, it is possible that they may experience well-being precisely because they reject most of the ideals of the paradigm.

Embracing Age: Aging Well in the Convent

While the nuns are engaged in American cultural practices and are indeed remarkably productive, independent, and happy in their old age, their understandings of personhood, temporality, individual agency and control, and productivity contrast with Western models. I suggest that the reasons the nuns report such remarkable well-being at the end of life may be tied to practices that contradict the premises behind the successful aging paradigm. The nuns' experiences of well-being may be enhanced precisely because they do not uphold the ideals of individual agency, productivity, independence, and permanent personhood.

I will walk through each of these cultural values to demonstrate how differently they emerge in the convent. Instead of valuing individual agency and control, the nuns value acceptance instead of independence; teach interdependence instead of valuing productivity; reinforce the idea that it is more important to *be* good than *do* good; and value every life stage, including old age, rather than valuing only "ageless" adulthood. Instead of embracing the current popular antiaging model, the nuns embrace aging, accepting it as a natural progression of the life course. I hypothesize that it is their cultural paradigm, which I call *embracing aging,* that sustains their health and well-being as they grow older.

Individual Agency, Control, and Acceptance

One of the central tenets of successful aging is the notion that each individual is responsible for her own health and well-being as she ages and that she should want and desire this responsibility (Lamb 2014, Lamb, Robbins-Ruszkowski, and Corwin 2017). The concept that each of us is and should be in control of their own body and future is a deeply ingrained American value. For most people in the United States, this type of individual agency is seen as a fundamental right and its desirability is rarely questioned in mainstream discourses. Decisions about one's health care, housing, and diet, for example, are seen as up to the individual. Individuals expect to be in charge of the decisions concerning where they live and what they eat, and physicians often make recommendations that patients are responsible for choosing to enact.

The nuns have a different understanding of agency and control. The vow of obedience, one of the three vows they take, is interpreted in the convent to have two meanings. First, they must be obedient to the divine, who is understood to hold the ultimate authority and power in their lives. Second, they must be obedient to institutional authorities, from the novice mistress who oversees them in their first few years in the convent, to the convent superiors who for much of their lives are responsible for decisions from the minute to the profound. In the first few years, the novice mistresses dictates minutiae in the nuns' everyday lives; after they leave the novitiate, institutional authorities continue to determine the details of their lives, such as what and when they eat, where they live and work, who they can socialize with, and when they can retire. Although the major institutional changes that followed Vatican II in the 1960s and 1970s have changed the meaning of obedience and have given many nuns more freedom to determine the details of their daily lives, the sisters have nevertheless lived much of their lives under strict institutional authority—an authority that is designed to strip the nuns of their sense of ego and independence, to deny them individual agency and control, and to "empty them of the self" in order to strengthen their sense of divine authority and love (Mensch 2005, 65; see also Clifford 2004 and Stetler 2012).

I suggest that it is this lack of agency and control that in fact supports the Sisters of the Sacred Heart as they age. Throughout their lives, the sisters have been encouraged to accept all decisions made for them with serenity and peace. My ethnographic data show that when they reach old age they understand illness and death as inevitable and meet these, too, with acceptance, serenity, and a sense of peace rather than with the feelings of failure, discouragement, or frustration many other North Americans report experiencing (Fisher 2014, 30). For example, when I met Sister Mary Bernard, she was ninety-eight years old. I was in my twenties, but I could barely keep up with her; she rushed down the hallways, greeting everyone in her path. She had a close relationship with God and spoke to me with great enthusiasm and humility about her happy childhood, her loving parents, her decades as a primary school teacher, and her enduring gratitude for what she saw as the many blessings in her life. The next year, at ninety-nine, Sister Mary Bernard was told that she needed to have her leg amputated above the knee. When I spoke to her about her impending surgery, she said, "You have to accept what God gives you. I'm still remembering that. The hardest thing is to accept the difficult things, but you know He loves you the most with those, because He's asking you to go through that for Him."

After the surgery, Sister Mary Bernard continued to live an active social life, holding court from her wheelchair in the hallways of the convent infirmary. She confessed that although she had thought she would not be able to live without her leg, "I accepted what God gave me." She told me that her faith had carried her though the surgery and continued to buoy her. During the time I spent in the convent, I witnessed many sisters encountering difficult medical news; though coming to terms with illness, pain, or physical decline was never easy for any of them, the majority of the nuns seemed to accept the changes in their physical bodies with remarkable equanimity.

It seems that the nuns' sense that divine and institutional authorities were in control and had power over their lives helped to relieve them from the responsibility of feeling they must exert control themselves. The years of practice in accepting that they did not have complete individual agency and control over their everyday lives seemed to help the sisters accept change as they aged.

Independence versus Interdependence

A second theme in the successful aging paradigm is the ideal of independence. Most of the research and popular books on successful aging presume that individuals value independence throughout their lives and would like to maintain it into old age (Lamb, Robbins-Ruszkowski, and Corwin 2017, 7). Dependence on others is seen not only as undesirable but as a moral failing.

When the nuns joined the convent, they made a distinct move away from a life of independence and committed themselves to a lifetime of communal living. They ate, slept, and bathed in shared spaces; they prayed together, worked together, and had to negotiate all aspects of everyday life with the other women in their community. There was little emphasis placed on independence and tremendous value placed on communal living, sharing, living in harmony, and serving others.

The nuns in the infirmary spent much of their time serving others and each other. During my first summer in the convent, I watched two sisters who lived in the infirmary take a walk together, arm in arm, each evening after supper around the beautiful grounds of the convent. One of the nuns was struggling with Alzheimer's disease and the other had painful arthritis that restricted her mobility. Sister Noella, who lived with Alzheimer's disease, was concerned that Sister Agatha, whose arthritis usually confined her to the infirmary, would not get any fresh air without her help, so she helped her physically navigate the hallway, the elevator, and the paths around the convent grounds. But Sister Agatha did not see the interaction in quite the same way; each evening she mustered the energy to overcome the limitations of her body to guide and orient Sister Noella so that she would not get lost on her walk around the convent grounds. Each sister made sure the other made it outside for a nightly stroll; the convent ethos of community and service allowed them each to see the walk as a way to serve the other. They did not speak about "dependence." Rather, each saw herself not as the one being helped, but as a friend putting herself second in order to serve another sister. Care was mutual and mutually enriching.

Although the North American antiaging paradigm places great value on the ability to live and function independently, epidemiological findings suggest that there are, in fact, strong correlations between living in a community and successful aging (Snowdon 2001). My own research confirms that the sisters' strong sense of community, mutuality, and shared life supported them as they aged. If the nuns declined in older age and were no longer able to function independently, they could draw on a lifetime of experience living interdependently and did not interpret dependence on others as moral failure; it was instead seen positively, as a way to serve and to be served.

Productivity and Being Good

A third theme in the successful aging paradigm is the pursuit of "active aging," the maintenance of productive activity into late life. This includes the maintenance of physical activity—for example, the ability to walk and exercise. It also includes the ability to remain a "productive" citizen, contributing to one's community into old age.

The nuns' community values informed how they understood the notion of productivity. Their vow of poverty required that they turned any savings they may have started out with, and all earnings, over to the convent. They were given a stipend to cover monthly expenses, such as toiletries, small purchases like books, and the occasional meal on the road, but all earnings were intended to symbolically and materially serve the community as a whole. The convent community emphasized the value of service through action. The nuns' work was evaluated based on whether it did good in the world. While the material contributions the nuns made from their salaries were valuable to the community in that they kept the convent operational, there was little relationship between the nuns' earning power and their sense of productive contribution. The nuns did value each other's material work, and when they retired, the sisters often had a hard time giving up positions in which they had been able to work and serve others. Yet the community made clear, especially to older sisters, that *being* good was just as important, if not more important, than *doing* good. When the nuns returned home to the convent to retire, they were met by a community of peers who reinforced the idea that being in community and praying was just as important as serving others through physical work. The nuns went to great effort to communicate that the work the elderly sisters did by praying was as important, if not more so, than the physical work they were doing or had done.

Sister Regina spoke to me about a transition in her life when she began to understand that being a good person was as or more important than being productive. She explained that she went through a spiritual transformation in which she stopped valuing the things she did and began to value the way she lived. Echoing American cultural values that equate productivity and morality,[7] she said that initially what was most important to her was doing or accomplishing things in the world—in other words, being productive: "I *did*—or, I say, I *do'd*—from the time I was able to do things until I was about—I must've been in my early forties. . . . The biggest thing was doing. That was my biggest prayer."

This sense that work in the world can be a form of prayer is a common Franciscan formulation. Sister Regina went on to note, however, that the productive accomplishment of things, even routinized prayer, became less and less meaningful as she grew older: "And so, it got to the point when I was in my forties that that didn't really mean anything to me. I did it because it was part of the protocol. . . . But being is harder than doing. And so, I've been being for a long time. For a long time. But the levels of being, they have become intensified, you know, I don't have to—I don't have to call God. God is part of who I am." As Sister Regina matured in her spirituality, she became more interested in *being*—or, as she defined it here, being with God. This transformation exemplified the convent's emphasis on valuing who a person was rather than what she had accomplished.

Because the nuns did not associate work with their material livelihood, and because they valued being good as equal to or above doing good, they did not seem to suffer a significant reduction in their sense of self-worth as they aged. When retiring or infirm nuns did experience concerns about their ability to serve others or make productive contributions to the community, they were met with enormous support from the other sisters, who again emphasized the importance of being good rather than doing good. The practice of thanking older sisters for their prayers was evidence of this; these expressions of gratitude for their prayers also demonstrated the importance the nuns placed on being in a relationship with God, something they could practice at any stage of life. Productivity in the convent was not necessarily tied to physical activity or material earnings. Instead the nuns were encouraged to experience themselves as valuable persons both during and after their materially productive and physically active years.

Permanent Personhood and Embracing Aging

The fourth theme in the successful aging paradigm is that of maintaining agelessness or permanent personhood. This involves "a vision of the ideal person as not really aging at all in later life, but rather maintaining the self of one's earlier years, while avoiding or denying processes of decline and conditions of oldness" (Lamb, Robbins-Ruszkowski, and Corwin 2017, 11; see also Lamb 2014). This vision associates personhood with competent active adulthood. In this paradigm children are seen as incomplete adults, on their way toward full personhood while older individuals are seen as moving away from full person-hood toward death or the end of personhood. Those who cannot function pro-ductively and competently in a capitalist setting—namely, children and elderly and disabled people—are segregated from engagement in everyday interaction (Kittay 2010; Rogoff 2003). Children in the United States are routinely seg-regated from engagement in the important or valued activities of adulthood, such as productive work and often even household chores, gaining access to these activities only when they become adults (Coppens et al. 2018; Paradise and Rogoff 2009). Similarly, disabled individuals are systematically separated from many everyday interactions where they may be seen as "disruptions." These patterns run in contrast to those of many other communities around the world, where all individuals are collaboratively involved in everyday household and production activities (Paradise and Rogoff 2009). Research in nursing homes and continuing care retirement communities has found that when individuals begin to display cognitive or physical decline, they experience exclusion from existing social networks.

Many retirement and continuing care institutions house individuals need-ing varying levels of care. But in the majority of these spaces in the United States, when individuals move from independent living to the assisted living or skilled nursing facilities—often only a few yards away—they find themselves stigmatized and abandoned by the other members of their former social net-works who are still living in the independent portion of the facility (Gross 2011; Shippee 2009). As Jane Gross, who writes about the social dynamics in con-tinuing care facilities, notes, "I visited only one congregate living environment for the elderly where I saw no stigma or social isolation among the more infirm, and that was the mother house [in a convent]—essentially a Continuing Care Retirement Community for aging nuns" (2011, 309). Sisters who were declin-ing and approaching death continued to be included as integral members of the community.

This pattern connects not only to the nuns' sense of community but also to their sense of what it means to be a valuable person. Unlike their secular peers, Christians exist in a temporal landscape that provides a notion of life after death (Robbins 2007). Death is not seen as an end point; rather, it is a transition from corporeality into another mode of being, a continuation of life in heaven. For the nuns I lived with, death was understood to be a passage or transformation rather than an end or, even, as in the antiaging paradigm, a failure. As such, in the convent, personhood and the values associated with it were not tied to pro-ductive adulthood. Rather, personhood was located within the soul, which was seen to begin before birth, at conception, and to endure after death, in heaven.

This view of personhood impacted how the nuns treated themselves and each other as they grew older. I observed that the expectation of life after death

seemed to reduce the nuns' fear of death. The idea that each individual continued to be a dignified person even after physical decline was evidenced in the
ways that the nuns treated each other as they aged. The sisters in the infirmary—
even those experiencing significant physical and mental decline—continued
to be meaningfully engaged in everyday activities. They continued to involve
their infirm peers in religious activities, at meals, and in social activities such
as card games. Even when their peers were not able to move or converse as they
had as younger adults, the other nuns continued to engage them in meaningful interactions as valuable persons until the end of life. Chapter 4 will document in more detail how the sisters engaged individuals with significant physical
and communicative decline in meaningful interaction.

Summary: Embracing Aging

The nuns may be heralded as "successes" within the contemporary aging paradigm, which is based on the cultural ideals of independence, productivity, and
permanent personhood and idealizes independence, physical health, individual control, and agency. Yet an examination of the nuns' lived experiences
demonstrates that the values they uphold run in contrast to the tenets of this
antiaging paradigm. In fact, their experiences with physical and mental well-
being may be supported by the fact that they embrace aging. In the nuns' cultural paradigm, they practice acceptance instead of valuing individual agency
and control. Over their lifetimes, they learn to accept that the divine and institutional authority hold ultimate authority in their lives. This understanding
that they are not in control of their lives helps the nuns cope with and accept
physical and mental decline, as well as death. Because the nuns live in community, the value of independence is not seen to be as important as interdependence. From the time they joined the convent, the nuns have had to learn to
spend their lives coordinating everyday tasks with others. This lifelong practice of interdependence seems to have supported the nuns as they transition
into the dependence that often accompanies physical decline. Activities that
involve reliance on others at the end of life can be interpreted as ways of serving and being served and can be more easily accepted by the nuns. Dependence, therefore, is understood not as a failure of individual autonomy, but as
a way to be served after a lifetime of serving others. The sisters may struggle
with the desire to continue to serve others, but being served is not a failure of
independence; it is a transition into a socially valued role.

Similarly, as members of a religious community who have taken vows of poverty, the nuns are not directly engaged in an economy that values production.
Indeed, they worked as nurses, teachers, and church administrators, and this
work was valued for how it impacted others and whether it made positive

changes in the world. And while this type of service could be valued for its productivity, the nuns also receive a significant amount of socialization that values *being* good over *doing* good. Through everyday practices and overt socialization, the nuns focus on being kind, peaceful, and generous and on loving people who had positive relationships with others and with the divine. (In chapter 3 we will return to the idea that socialization is a process that continues throughout the life course.) Finally, the nuns see personhood as located in the soul rather than the embodied person. This means that valued personhood is not limited to productive adulthood. A person's value extends in time before birth (beginning at conception) and beyond death into the afterlife. This sense that individuals are valuable members of the community even when they are not productive adults encourages the nuns to treat others in the community with respect, dignity, and engagement even when they display significant cognitive and physical decline.

As we look closely at the cultural values associated with aging in the convent, it becomes clear that it would be inaccurate to claim that the health outcomes that the nuns experience are connected to the cultural values promoted in the successful aging paradigm. It seems that instead of the values promoted in this antiaging paradigm, the nuns' model of interdependence—being rather than doing good, valuing people whether or not they are productive citizens, and embracing decline—supports them as they age.

If we present independent, productive agelessness as "success," an achievement that one can earn through hard work, it inadvertently shames and blames those individuals who by no fault of their own encounter pain, chronic conditions, and death. When we remember that many of these chronic conditions correlate with environmental factors that disproportionately impact lower-income communities and people of color in the United States, this also reveals a major social justice issue (see, for example, Donohoe 2012; Margai 2013).

While positive health outcomes are undoubtedly desirable, it is not only potentially emotionally distressing but also inaccurate to adopt a model that stigmatizes decline. Sarah Lamb and others have suggested that, as a replacement, Americans might do well to adopt a model that includes *meaningful* decline, and I agree that this would be a helpful paradigm shift away from the current antiaging model. I propose that exploration of cultural paradigms like the nuns' embrace of aging allow us to begin to imagine alternatives to the current mainstream model.

The following chapters will delve more deeply into how the nuns have learned to accept aging and decline and how they have come to experience their aging bodies. Their model of embracing aging is a culturally specific one, and my goal is to show readers why and how the nuns experience such positive health outcomes. I hope that, as this book progresses, readers appreciate the delicate and complex cultural practices, ideologies, and histories that have come together to shape the moment in time in which these sisters live in and the complex unfolding that has shaped their aging experience.

As with all cultural models, the nuns' model is not better than others, and I hope that no reader takes this chapter or the book as a whole to be proscriptive. The book seeks to shed light on how and why the nuns age the way they do, but the answer comes as a deeply intertwined, habitually instantiated set of cultural practices that have unfolded over lifetimes. As always, explorations of cultural practices and models that are different from one's own can be illuminating—showing us both what is foreign to us and what is familiar as new perspectives allow us to see ourselves in new ways.

While I suggest that it is essential not to conflate the cultural values associated with the successful aging paradigm with a universal scientific "truth" (as it is often represented in the literature), I would similarly caution the reader against concluding that the nuns' model could be applied wholesale outside its context. My hope is that—rather than replacing the current model—this chapter has provided evidence that there can be multiple models of aging rather than one "successful" one and, more important, that it is possible to embrace aging and flourish in the process.

3

Talking to God

• •

Prayer as Social Support

It was 2:00 p.m. on a hot July afternoon. The convent outside was abuzz with life; the sticky, humid air hummed with insects and birds. Inside the great brick convent walls, I followed Sister Irma down the hallway. At eighty, she walked with a slight limp. She had a thick apron tied around her waist and held a bottle of lotion in one hand. Inside the infirmary, the air was so cool that I began to feel goose bumps develop on my forearms.

I followed Sister Irma into room after room. The afternoon light streamed in the windows, and she greeted each of her elderly peers with a hello that was often followed by a playful tease or joke. She then sat down to offer each sister a foot massage. Every day since she had retired from a lifetime of teaching and working in a rural parish, Sister Irma spent her afternoons like this—walking down the infirmary hallways and massaging the feet of her elderly sisters. As she massaged, the nuns gabbed, reminiscing about the past, gossiping about who was doing what, and checking in on what each of them had been up to that week.

In one of the rooms, under a handmade yellow and brown afghan, one sister reclined on a medical bed with her eyes closed. She moaned quietly and made no indication that she was aware of our presence next to her bed. Sister Irma cupped the sister's knobby hand in her warm palms and introduced me to Sister Dominique. She then drew the sign of the cross on Sister Dominique's forehead and said to her, "Thank you for your prayers. Your family and our community are grateful for your prayers." She softly lay down Sister Dominique's hand on top of the afghan and we moved on down the hallway.

We cannot know what Sister Dominique experienced, but this moment and others like it tell us how important prayer was in the community. If Sister Dominique could hear Sister Irma, she was reminded that even as she lay in her room, her prayers, defined in the community as any verbal or nonverbal form of communion with God, were valuable. In her bed, moaning, she was told that she was valuable, meaningful; she was just where she was meant to be.

A growing literature has found that prayer seems to have remarkable benefits for those who routinely engage in it, contributing to physical and psychological well-being (Carlson, Bacaseta, and Simanton 1988; Koenig 2003; Lim and Putman 2010; Salsman et al. 2005). In his research with nuns, David Snowdon has suggested that prayer, which his epidemiological study does not directly measure, has as a strong impact on quality of life (2001, 202). This chapter will look at how the language of prayer—and specifically one type of prayer, the petition (also called intercessory prayer)—functions in the convent and how it impacts the nuns' experiences in the world as they age.

In chapter 2 we learned that prayer was a mode through which older sisters who were infirm could continue to contribute to the convent. This chapter dives deeper into the workings of prayer to explore what prayer achieves for the nuns in the convent. Before looking directly at prayer, it is important to revisit how linguistic anthropologists see language. Language is not merely representational; it does more than represent or describe things in the world. Language also has a far more complex and dynamic role in human experience and interaction. As J. L. Austin asserts in *How to Do Things with Words* (1962), language can do things in the world. Language can also do multiple things simultaneously. For example, linguistic anthropologist Greg Urban, who has studied ritual wailing in Amerindian Brazil, has found that the ritual wailing that accompanies displays of grief at separations or after death functions in two ways. First, the wailing functioned as a way for individuals to express emotions—in this case, sadness or grief as they found themselves separated by space or by death from their loved ones. Second, wailing has a performative function, as "a covert expression for the desire for sociability" (Urban 1988, 385). In other words, the wailing was not only an expression of an emotion or set of emotions but also functioned to express a desire for social connection in that particular moment. Charles Briggs, a linguistic and medical anthropologist who has also written about wailing in South America, has similarly suggested that Warao ritual wailing can function as a way for social ties or "closeness" to be both performed and constructed through the wailing process (Briggs 1993, 931). In both cases, language is emotionally expressive and functions to create or maintain social bonds between people.

This chapter builds on a model of language in which language is understood to function on multiple levels at once. Prayer, like ritual wailing, is a ritual in which individuals communicate with the divine through ritually proscribed linguistic forms. Like ritual wailing, prayer can function as an emotional expression, communicating, for example, gratitude, love, or sadness. I will suggest that, like ritual wailing, it can also function as a call for sociality. In intercessory prayer, or petitions, the nuns solicit the divine to intercede in the world. These prayers include petitions for God to help those who are ill or to assist those in need. While I was in the convent, I recorded 144 petitions that were spoken during Mass or during smaller group prayer meetings.[1] The prayers were part of a particular ritual sequence that began with an opening in which the priest at Mass or a member of the prayer group cued the petitions. Following the recitation of each petition, the speaker cued the closure of the prayer with a statement indicating the end of the petition such as "We pray" or "For this we pray," at which point the community recited together "Lord, hear our prayer." This sequence was then repeated until the end of the set of petitions.

This chapter suggests that petitions functioned in the convent in a number four ways: as a mode to request help from the divine, as a way to index the presence of God, as a form of social support, and finally as a way to socialize sisters into how to approach the end of life and death.

I should point out to the reader that the analysis of prayer in this chapter builds from my training as a linguistic anthropologist. When I am analyzing language closely, I transcribe the interactions recorded in my data using transcription conventions typical of the field. The transcription conventions in linguistic anthropology divide the transcript by line and include a level of detail often left out of block quotations. The transcription conventions appear in the appendix. The act of transcription is a theoretical act in which the researcher decides what to include on the page, how to encode it in text, and what to leave out (Ochs 1979). If you are new to linguistic anthropology, I encourage you to attend to the detail with curiosity and patience. In doing so you will find that meaning making occurs not only in the words spoken but also in the pauses, silences, and false starts, as well as in the prosody, pitch, and embodied gestures and movements that accompany the spoken word.

Prayer as a Way to Request Help from the Divine

Petitions in the convent functioned most obviously as a way to ask the divine to intercede in the world. The nuns understood that while there were ways in which they could act in the world, there were also limits to what they could achieve as humans. God, on the other hand, had the capacity to act in the world in ways that reached beyond human limits. The nuns also understood God to be all powerful and responsive to prayers. Kurt Bruder has written that blessings are "invocations of divine favor" (1998, 466) on an activity or individual and, as such, when someone recites a blessing that person is speaking directly to the divine, petitioning God to bless the recipient. Petitions as well as blessings are requests that God might or might not fulfill. Nevertheless, the nuns viewed intercessory prayers as a way to do something good in the world; by asking the divine to intercede in the world, they saw themselves as helping to create positive action on earth.

The idea that prayer is a way to petition the divine to act in the world is an ontological claim. It is a claim about what exists in the world and what is real that has implications for what counts as reality in the nuns' lives. That God could intervene and that the nuns' prayers could inspire that intervention is a claim about the fundamental makeup of reality. I, personally, did not grow up with this type of orientation toward the world or toward prayer. I almost never witnessed anyone in my family pray, and when they did—for instance, when lighting the Hanukkah candles—it was a routine that had symbolic meaning but not practical implications. The nuns' orientation to a world where the divine could intervene contrasts with this. Let us take this prayer, for instance:

EXAMPLE 1: PETITION FOR GOOD WEATHER

<u>Participants</u>

SI: Sister Irene
ALL: Congregants in chapel during Mass

```
01 SI:   For good? weather and good crops this season
02       (0.3) we pray.
03       (0.2)
04 ALL: Lord hear our prayer.
```

The fact that this prayer was recited aloud demonstrates that the nuns felt they could do something to care for their neighbors and the families who made their livelihood through farming. The prayer was a form of care and a way to act in the world.

When I was in the convent, many of the sisters told me, in separate interactions, about a podiatrist who came to the infirmary on a regular basis to care for the older sisters' feet. The podiatrist had been married for years but, to her great sadness, had not been able to conceive a child. She asked the sisters to pray for her to have children. In each of the renditions of the story, it ended in nearly the same way: "So the next year, she had twins, a boy and a girl." I heard this story many times and, each time, the sisters matter-of-factly and sometimes quite proudly recounted the community's impact on the podiatrist's conception of her twins. A few of the sisters even joked that they prayed "too well"—hence the twins.

This ontological orientation toward the world likely had psychological effects. The practice of praying every day to a God who the nuns *knew* loved them, and the practice of habitually engaging in an act they saw as positively impacting the world must have shaped their experience in the world. The nuns spoke about this practice as an experience of God's love.

A number of studies have found that having a sense of purpose is a key contributor to well-being in old age, and, as Patrick Hill, Grant Edmonds, and Sarah Hampson write, "has been consistently linked to subjective and objective health markers" (2017, 1; see also Windsor, Curtis, and Luszcz 2015). Similarly, having a sense that one is not solely in charge of the good and bad outcomes of the future may have also had positive outcomes on the nuns' stress levels, as well as their sense of comfort and support; as we saw in chapter 2, the nuns reported high rates of social support.

This first function of prayer, a request to God to intervene, may itself be a process that brought the sisters comfort as it reinforced the idea that God can and does act in the world. It was also a way in which they could feel that they had achieved an outcome in the world, such as in the case of the collective prayers for the podiatrist's pregnancy.

Prayer as a Way to Index the Presence of the Divine

Because God is invisible, interaction with and devotion to the divine provides a unique conundrum that distinguishes it from other types of interaction. When interacting with God, the nuns were engaged with an invisible interlocutor who, in anthropologist Tanya Luhrmann's words, "gives none of the ordinary signs of existence" (2012, xi). When interacting with copresent humans, communication is usually met with verbal or embodied responses such as a nod or eye gaze or with discourse markers such as "oh" or "mm-hmm." When the nuns prayed together at Mass or in small groups, God did not show any of the typical signs of conversational uptake. There was no nod, no "mm-hmm," no eye gaze from the divine.

As with other forms of religious language, the invisibility of a divine interlocutor shapes the way in which the communication unfolds. For example, in the petitions I recorded in the convent, 65 percent of them addressed the divine by name: alternately "Lord," "God," or "Christ." These terms served to call on God and to publicly perform to the audience at Mass or in the prayer group who was being addressed; it was as if the speakers were routinely reminding the group (and/or the divine) that God was the one being prayed to. In addition, the prayers included the ritually repeated "We pray" and the ritual refrain

"Lord, hear our prayer," which called attention to the act that was being performed as it was performed. This is metapragmatic, meaning that the act being performed (prayer) was publicly announced as it was taking place (through the words "We pray"). As I have written elsewhere, this metapragmatic affirmation of the action of prayer "confirms the collective will and collective desire to engage in the prayer" (Corwin 2014, 183).

This linguistic structure affirmed the existence of the divine in two ways. First, as the speaker performed the petition, asking the divine to intercede, she was making public to the community her understanding that the divine was present, listening, and could intercede in the world. Second, as the audience joined in the speech act by reciting "For this we pray" in unison, they, too, affirmed the divine's presence or possible presence. Through this performative act the divine—an invisible interlocutor who, unlike material beings, could not be publicly seen or heard—was indexed, or pointed to, as present and as a viable recipient of prayer by all of the parties participating in the prayer. Petitions, therefore, functioned to confirm the existence and presence of the divine for participants, rendering an invisible interlocutor publicly available for communication. In simpler terms, by routinely announcing that they were praying to God, the nuns were communicating that God, while invisible, was available to be spoken to.

This process is an example of the coconstruction of the lived world. There is something quite powerful about the collective ratification of a divine but invisible interlocutor; it has the potential to make the divine's presence and existence feel more real to those present. For example, Susan Harding, an atheist researcher who worked with evangelical Christians who were following Rev. Jerry Falwell, writes about an incident in which she interviewed a man who—rather than answering the questions Harding posed—had "witnessed" to her, attempting to convert her to Christianity. Harding writes that as she drove home that evening, she just barely avoided being involved in a car accident. As she reeled from almost being hit, she found herself wondering, "What is God trying to tell me?" Harding interprets this experience as the process of acquiring a new language, the language of the Christians she had been spending her days studying (2000, 32, 34). This anecdote demonstrates how even without consciously attempting to adapt to a cultural community, the habituated practices of the community members one spends time with can become entrained in one's habits and practices.

Harding's moment of speaking and thinking like the community she was researching did not, of course, produce an enduring transformation; Harding did not become Christian. As Luhrmann, who also studies evangelical Christians, suggests, the process of learning to become part of a culture in which people hear and talk to God encompasses a dynamic, embodied learning process involving both the body and emotional entrainment (Luhrmann 2004,

2012). Through Harding's anecdote we begin to see how our lived world and ontological realities are coconstructed with our environment; over time, individuals are shaped by the habituated practices that they engage in as members of a cultural community, As the sisters collectively spoke to the divine, these habituated practices shaped their language and their experiences of the divine. Harding's moment of communion with God did not last, but for Catholics for whom the divine has always been an enduring presence, the collective indexing of his presence no doubt renews this experience. As such, the words of a petition could render God more present for the nuns.

Prayer as Social Support

Returning to the concept at the start of the chapter that ritual lament can communicate a desire for sociability, I found that in the convent prayer could often function as a form of sociability, a way for the nuns to communicate not only with God but also with each other. As petitions for God to intervene in the world on behalf of others, their prayers were seen by the nuns as a direct form of social support. The sisters were actively involved in serving their peers as well as the local community—for example, providing physical care, pastoral care, running food pantries, and working for social justice. When they encountered needs in the world that they could not resolve themselves—for example, a drought impacting farmers—the nuns turned to intercessory prayer to ask the divine for aid. In this way, the petitions functioned as additional social support they offered their community.

This is not the only way in which the petitions functioned as a form of social support in the convent. When I analyzed the petitions, I found that many of them provided information that would be extraneous if the petitions were directed only to God. The God to whom the sisters were addressing in their prayers was understood to be omniscient or all knowing, yet the nuns provided a myriad of details in their petitions that an omniscient God would not need. For example, in the following petition, Sister Marie prayed for Sister Laura Mantle, who was ill:

EXAMPLE 2: PETITION FOR SISTER LAURA MANTLE
Participants
SM: Sister Marie
ALL: Group of seven nuns and the author

01 SM: And (then prayer uh) special for Sister Laura
02   Mantle, who's
03   back up in the third floor a' Saint Anthony
04   Ha:ll (.)
05   um, her blood pressure

```
06      spiked right after lunch an' (1.5)
07      They wouldn't even tell 'er what it wa:s
08      (1.0) u:m (2.0)
09      Thank God, (.)
10      God who would give her um (1.0) grace,
11      (2.0)
12      and she asks—asked for the grace to accept
13      what (3.0)
14      she i:s dealing with.
15      For Sister Laura we pray=
16 ALL: =Lord hear our prayer.
```

In this excerpt, Sister Marie provided a tremendous amount of information, specifying not only the first and last name of the person for whom she was praying but also where she was located, what happened to her, and when it happened. She provided a narrative including detailed background information as a prelude to her prayer. Only after listing these details did she ask God to provide grace for Sister Laura to accept her current condition.

Philosopher of language Paul Grice has outlined a number of conversational norms now known as Grice's Maxims. The conversational maxim of quantity states that people expect each other to "make [their] contribution as informative as is required (for the current situation)" and "not make [their] contribution more informative than is required" (Grice 1989, 26). Violating the maxim of quantity could involve answering a question with less information than is necessary—for example, if one person asked another, "Can you tell me what time it is?" and the person responded, "Yes." This response would accurately answer the question about whether or not the person *can* tell the person the time, but it fails to make the contribution as informative as required by failing to report the time. Similarly, if someone asked, "Can you tell me what time it is?" and their interlocutor replied "It is 9:00 a.m. here, and noon in New York, and Greenwich Mean Time is currently 5:00 p.m.," this would also violate the maxim of quantity by providing more information than necessary. In typical everyday interaction, most speakers avoid violating the maxims. Deliberately violating a maxim—for example, as a joke or to antagonize someone—is referred to as "flouting the maxim." My son does this, but even as a child he is quite aware of how annoying it is; in fact, that is precisely why he finds it so funny to do.

There is no reason to assume that Sister Marie and the other sisters who provide much more information than God would need are flouting the maxim of quantity. When I clarified with Sister Rita whether the nuns believe that God knows the worldly details such as what floor or what room a person is in, she laughed and responded, "If He doesn't, we're in a bad way," confirming that these details would not be necessary for God to hear before he could answer intercessory prayers (Corwin 2014, 183).

If God was omniscient, and already knew who Sister Laura Mantle was, where she lived, and what happened after lunch when her blood pressure spiked, then why would Sister Marie include this information in her prayer? If we assume that she and the other sisters are not in a habit of regularly flouting Grice's Maxims, then Sister Marie must have included this information for a reason. If we "zoom out," so to speak, on the prayer interaction, we begin to see this prayer differently. At Mass, when a sister recited a petition, she stood at a podium to the left of the altar, facing wooden pews filled with her peers and a handful of community members who attended Mass with the sisters. During evening prayers, a sister reciting her petition faced a circle of chairs filled with other sisters. If we imagine that Sister Marie's intercessory prayer was directed only to God, then these sisters would be seen merely as an audience to the prayer. In fact, the sisters hearing Sister Marie's prayer were women who knew Sister Laura Mantle, who lived in her community in or near Saint Anthony Hall. They knew many nuns named Sister Laura, but only one Sister Laura Mantle on the third floor of Saint Anthony Hall. If we imagine that this prayer was designed not only for God but also for these sisters, then the inclusion of this detailed information not only does not violate Grice's maxim of quantity but in fact would have been quite useful.

If we see the prayers as directed not only to the divine, but also to the copresent interlocutors, the sisters in the room, the function of the prayer expands. The sisters listening to this prayer now knew which Sister Laura was being prayed for. They learned where she was, that she had been moved to Saint Anthony Hall on the third floor of the convent infirmary, what had happened, and that she was suffering. This information enabled the sisters to visit Sister Laura, to comfort her, and to provide any assistance that she might need. In other words, the petitions, while directed to the divine, also functioned as a way for the sisters to learn what social support was needed in the convent. The sisters in the room where Sister Marie recited her prayer might not have known about Sister Laura's condition, but after hearing the prayer they could visit her and provide support or comfort. Intercessory prayer therefore functioned as a means to communicate needs to both God and the community so that the sisters could provide social and spiritual support for each other.

Petitions are a channel of communication that are a particularly efficient method to convey needs to many people at once; at Mass petitions reached the entire community. The prayers therefore allowed for direct communication of needs to a community that had the capacity to act in the world. Following Mass, at meals, I often heard the sisters talking about how people were doing, who had been visiting whom, and who needed care. The petition might communicate a need, and individuals after Mass would follow up by checking in with those closest to the person whose need had been named, checking in with a nurse, or simply walking to up to a room to check in on the sister. In this way the prayers functioned not only through God but also through the nuns themselves.

The petitions also functioned as a way to communicate care and support to someone who was in the room. For instance, in the following excerpt Sister Irma prayed for me and my family during an evening prayer meeting. At the time, I was six months pregnant with my daughter.

EXAMPLE 3: PETITION FOR THE AUTHOR
Participants
SI: Sister Irma
ALL: Four nuns and the author

```
01 SI:  For little baby girl, cradled in her mother's womb,
02      that she can come to be healthy and happy as,
03      as one of us.
04      For her mommy and her dad and her little brother,
05      her big brother.
06 ALL: For this we pray.
```

In this prayer, Sister Irma embedded a number of intercessions: first for the health and happiness of my unborn daughter, and then for me, the mother, and for my partner and our son, who was a one and a half years old at the time. While she was communicating directly with the divine, asking God to provide for our health and well-being, it is important to note that I was copresent, a ratified listener to the prayer. In addition, when I spoke the words "For this we pray", I was also a speaker of the prayer. As I listened to and coproduced the prayer with Sister Irma, I heard that she cared for me and my family and that she was intervening on our behalf by asking the divine to provide for our health. The prayer functioned not only as a request to the divine but also as communication of social support to me as I heard her pray on my behalf. In this way petitions functioned as direct communication of social support to individuals who were in the room.

While these types of very personal prayers were more common in smaller prayer groups, there were also prayers for individuals during larger services in the chapel. For instance, the following prayer was spoken on behalf of the sisters celebrating their jubilee, the anniversary of those sisters' time in the convent.

EXAMPLE 4: PETITION FOR JUBILARIANS
Participants
SJ: Sister Josephine
ALL: Congregants in chapel during Mass

```
01 SJ:  We rejoice and give thanks for our jubilarians
02      for their faithful commitment in service within
03      the Catholic community (.)
04      and beyond.
05 ALL: For this we pray.
```

On the day Sister Josephine recited this petition, she looked out over pews filled with sisters and the families who had come to celebrate the jubilarians. This prayer not only functioned as a prayer of thanksgiving directed to God but also as a public acknowledgment of the lifetime of work each of the sisters had dedicated to the convent and the communities in which they worked. This public recognition was also a form of social support, displaying gratitude and acknowledgment for the sisters who had dedicated decades of their lives to service.

Prayer as Socialization

In her examination of narratives in Spanish-language Catholic religious education, or *doctrina*, classes, Patricia Baquedano-López (2000) describes how narratives are used as a mode of socialization, orienting children into shared history, shared identity, and "community moral order" (430, 441). Baquedano-López writes that through socialization in the *doctrina* classes, "individual and collective identities are constructed, maintained, and transformed vis-à-vis positionings within a web of moral expectations" (2000, 443). I have argued elsewhere that petitions are similarly embedded in an ethical framework. As public communication with God during the ritual of Mass or the Hours, these prayers encode guidance on how to act, how to feel, and how to be a "good" person in the convent community (Corwin 2014, 186).

Socialization, the process of learning to be a competent member of a cultural community, continues throughout the life course (Garrett and Baquedano-López 2002; Jacoby and Gonzales 1991; Schieffelin and Ochs 1986). Although most research on socialization has focused on childhood, socialization at the end of life has been shown to impact how individuals age and die. For instance, in a study of older adults approaching death, Holly Prigerson, a sociologist of medicine, has found that if a patient's caregiver does not accept death, the patient is not likely to come to terms with her own impending death (1992).

By publicly performing direction on how to be in the world, prayer can be a key mode of socialization. Psychologist Lisa Capps and linguistic anthropologist Elinor Ochs studied Euro-American children learning to pray in Sunday school and found that modeling behavior was a key form of socialization for the children as they engaged in the cultivation of a "prayerful attitude" and "a quiet way of being" (2001, 39, 45).

When we look at prayer as a form of socialization, we gain insight into the particular cultural values of aging in the convent. In chapter 2, I made the argument that the "successful aging" paradigm is a cultural model. I suggested that although this antiaging paradigm is often presented as a neutral scientific model, impartially describing findings on how people experience increased health and well-being as they age, the paradigm instead promotes American cultural ideals. Individuals within a particular cultural context are often unaware of the cultural values they foster in their own lives. This is the ethereal magic of culture: it undergirds almost all of what we do, but we are often profoundly unaware of its compelling power over how we move through our own world.

Socialization practices, in which individuals shape the cultural practices of members of their own group, can be a rich site at which to learn about the cultural values of a community. There are a number of excellent socialization studies that look at how infants and children learn to become fluent members of their cultural communities (see, for example, Berman 2019; Bock and Johnson 2004; Chapin 2014; Lancy 2015; Ochs and Izquierdo 2009; and Rogoff 2003). Since Elinor Ochs and Bambi Schieffelin introduced the notion of language socialization—that is, how individuals are socialized to language and through language—in 1984, there has been a growing literature on language socialization. Yet while most scholars agree that socialization occurs throughout the life course, there has been less research on the ways in which adults and older adults engage in socialization processes.

Prayers are one way in which the nuns were actively involved in producing and receiving messages about how to age. When something was chosen as a topic for an intercession, it was sanctioned by the speaker and the community as something that was *worth* praying for. Not everything was understood to be worth bringing to God to ask for intercession. For instance, the nuns would have thought it absurd to pray for something that an individual could easily achieve herself with some assistance, such as cleaning a room or lifting a heavy object. Instead, the sisters would simply ask another person for help. They might ask for the strength to endure something, but never for God to intervene in a task that they could accomplish themselves. Similarly, the nuns never asked for the divine to intervene on the body's healing process. For instance, if someone had fallen and broken a hip, the nuns did not lay hands on the person and ask God to heal the bone, or if someone had cancer, they did not ask for God to take away the cancer. In part, this has to do with the ideologies of pain and illness that will be discussed in chapter 6. The nuns also focused most of their prayers on intercessions for others. Only very rarely and in very specific formats, which will be discussed below, did they request intercessions for themselves. But how did the nuns learn what should be prayed for and what should not? Many evangelical Christians, for instance, pray for direct healing, for the divine to eliminate chronic illness or to heal conditions otherwise seen as incurable.

Some groups of Christians pray for material wealth for themselves, their families, and their communities. These types of petitions would be extremely unusual for Franciscans. Many of these practices are likely socialized when individuals are young. Most of the sisters grew up in Catholic households in which they would have encountered prayers at home, during Mass, and at Sunday school and would have become familiar with Catholic values, including humility, and practices such as praying for others rather than for oneself. On the other hand, learning how to approach the process of aging, chronic illness, and the end of life would have been new for most of the sisters in the convent. This was a process that the sisters engaged in only as adults or older adults.

As public communication about how the world should be or how the petitioner hoped it would be, petitions modeled ways to discuss aging and the end of life. The nuns' petitions did not ask for the process of aging, decline, or death to be altered; rather than praying for physical healing or avoidance of death, the petitions focused on acceptance, peace, optimism, and assuaging fear or anxiety about the end of life (see Corwin 2014, 187). The following petition, which asked for healing and acceptance for sisters in the infirmary, asked the divine for intercession on the sisters' behalf and gently oriented the audience, which included sisters in the infirmary, to how one should approach illness.

EXAMPLE 5: PETITION FOR HEALING AND ACCEPTANCE
Participants
SB: Sister Bernadette

01 SB: For healing and acceptance for
02   our sisters
03   in Saint Anthony Hall.
04   (1.3)
05   We pray.

This petition had the three functions I have outlined in the chapter thus far. First, the speaker, Sister Bernadette, asked the divine to provide for the sisters who were living in the convent infirmary. Second, the petition functioned as a form of social support. This prayer was spoken during Mass. Any of the sisters who could not attend Mass had the ability to tune in via the closed-circuit televisions installed in each of the rooms in the infirmary. On the occasions that I accompanied the sisters who brought Communion to their peers in Saint Anthony Hall who could not come downstairs for Mass, I saw that the majority of the rooms had the televisions on and tuned in to Mass. The majority of the sisters who lived in Saint Anthony Hall and those who might someday need to go to the infirmary wing were aware that the community was praying for them. Finally, this prayer functioned as a way to socialize the aging sisters into how a sister should approach aging, what she should strive for, and what to ask of God.

Just as the prayer for Sister Laura Mantle asked for her to be given the "grace to accept what she is dealing with," this prayer asked that the sisters in the infirmary be granted "acceptance" as they experienced illness and decline. Acceptance in the face of decline is a radically different project from what we see in popular discourse in the United States. In chapter 2 we saw that the current antiaging paradigm emphasizes practices that allow individuals to be healthy enough to live independently and to be active and productive for as long as possible. The prayers in the convent emphasized something quite different. The prayer here emphasized both healing and acceptance; that these two were requested together demonstrates a particular attitude toward aging and illness. Acceptance does not imply giving up, since healing (which may be physical or spiritual) implies a change and hope. On the other hand, healing was not the sole focus. That the prayer for healing was accompanied by a prayer for acceptance implied that healing was not the only goal. The attention to acceptance communicated that those who were infirm and approaching the end of life should strive for acceptance of their physical reality, whatever that might be.

Acceptance—and "grace," as we saw in the prayer for Sister Laura Mantle— were values that emerged prominently in the socialization process in the convent. While acceptance itself might not put an end to the condition an individual was experiencing, acceptance could alleviate a secondary source of suffering. Wishing to be out of pain or feeling angry that one is in pain can cause stress or negative psychological outcomes beyond the symptom of the pain itself. In addition to potentially reducing this second source of pain, socialization into acceptance also provided the sisters with an acknowledgment that the community was not asking them to be any different than they were.

The prayer in example 5 was structured such that God was asked to grant the individual acceptance of what she was experiencing. This prayer communicated to an individual who could not do what she used to do—perhaps she was bedridden and could no longer serve the community physically, or perhaps she was in pain or knew that she was dying—that she was just where God wanted her to be. The community had requested and therefore given their blessing for her to accept this. Rather than fretting that she should get better and serve the community or that she should recover and not be a burden to her caretakers, the prayer communicated that the morally sanctioned thing for a sister in the infirmary to do at that moment was to accept what she was experiencing.

When I tell people outside the convent that my research focuses on the question of why Catholic nuns experience well-being at the end of life, people often respond by joking that nuns are healthy because life in a convent involves less stress. Often I hear this expressed in the form of one of two jokes: "Well, of course they do! They don't have to take care of husbands!" or "They have no children to worry about! Of course they're healthier!" While these jokes might say more about how the individual feels about his or her own role as a spouse or parent than about the nuns, I often find myself explaining how hard the nuns work, how much they endure in service to their community, how much they once gave up in terms of self-determination, and how late into life they work. I do think, however, that these joking explanations that the nuns' well-being might have something to do with reduced stress have some truth to them. Yet the stress is not from any "freedom" from a spouse or children. The nuns, in fact, were beholden to many people in their community in ways that are as deeply entangled and were certainly no less trying than the entanglements of kinship. Instead I would suggest that it was the community's emphasis on acceptance and grace and the supportive mode through which this was communicated that reduced the nuns' stress as they aged. The nuns were encouraged not to focus on changing what they could not change; instead they were socialized to accept what they could not change through prayers that also communicated that they were cared for by their peers and by God.

The petitions socialized the sisters to accept not only illness and decline but also death. The following prayer, spoken during Mass, was offered for the dying.

EXAMPLE 6: PETITION FOR THE DYING
Participants
SC: Sister Christine

01 SC: For those near death,
02   that the promise and hope of eternal life may
03   bring them
04   comfort and consolation.
05   We pray to the Lord.

Before looking at the content of this prayer, I would like to point to the existence of the prayer itself. The fact that the topic of the prayer focused on death and acknowledged death and those who were approaching it is significant. That the topic was addressed in this public space, during Mass, is itself a socialization message that communicated that death was a culturally acceptable topic for discussion. Death was not hidden away or stigmatized, and this mirrors the dying process in the convent. As sisters declined and approached the end of life, they remained valued members of the community and continued to be integrated in the community in whatever way made sense for them as individuals.

This socialization process was ongoing. When the sisters retired from outside work and returned to the convent, they were each asked to fill out a packet of surveys that prompted them to describe their wishes for their death and funeral. The questions in the surveys included details such as whether they would prefer to have music playing or silence during their final days and hours and whether they would like many visitors or just one or two sisters. The surveys also asked the sisters to outline their preferences for their funeral Mass and burial. They could name whom they would like to have speak at their funeral and what passages they would like recited, and they could specify which type of casket they preferred out of a choice of three that included a minimalistic environmentally friendly choice. The fact that the sisters were asked to fill out these surveys communicated through an institutional socialization process that death and dying were important to think about, that dying was normal and natural, and that each nun should think through her own dying process. The consistent communication that death was normal, natural, and a worthy topic for prayer and conversation socialized the sisters into a particular orientation toward death—one that avoided stigma and promoted acceptance of the existence of death as a normal and universal process.

Returning to the prayer above, the way that death was spoken about is also relevant in understanding how the nuns were socialized into death and dying. The petition reminded those who were actively dying as well as those who were approaching the end of life that the community supported them. Dying was not seen as a failure or as something to be feared or avoided; it was a natural part of life that the community actively acknowledged and supported. The prayer also suggested that heaven and "eternal life" (line 02) offered comfort and consolation for those who might have been having a hard time transitioning from life to death.

The prayer therefore oriented the sisters to a particular ontological orientation to time and personhood, one that we will see Sister Carline discuss in chapter 6. Rather than a termination of life, death represented a transition of one type of life to another as life in heaven. The form life took might change as one shed the body, but death was not an end. Instead it was seen as a transition into eternal life in heaven. For the nuns, death was not something that needed to be feared; it was seen as a positive transition. M. Brooke Barss, a psychiatrist and Buddhist chaplain who worked with a community of Sisters of Mercy in Vermont, writes that she was surprised that the sisters she worked with did not see death as a difficult topic. She writes that when she questioned this lack of attention to death, "the sisters set me straight: for them death is a coming home to Christ. It doesn't frighten them at all, and indeed, death to this life seems to be a comforting prospect. For them, heaven is a place to be with God, and for many a promised reunion with loved ones. As one sister explained, 'Rejoining God in heaven is what it's all about: our service to others, our ministry and prayers, and tolerating the pain of this earthly existence, is working toward a coming home. We don't worry about death. We celebrate the coming home'" (Barss 2018, 37–38).

While most women who join a convent have the understanding that death is not an ending but rather a transition to heaven, the attitude of celebration expressed here is something that comes with years of cultural practice. Death, even for people who have been taught that they will go to heaven, can be scary. In the Franciscan Sisters of the Sacred Heart Convent, petitions offered an example of how this socialization process can occur. By modeling culturally appropriate behaviors, practices, and emotional states, the prayers offered, through socialization, an attitude of comfort and celebration. Through their content and design, the petitions modeled what attitudes were expected and what was normal and good. Through the focus on acceptance of suffering and decline together, the petitions modeled an ethos of humility, concern for others, and an ideal of embracing aging. This socialization process was further sustained when the nuns witnessed their peers grow older and die. Their dying peers were not hidden away, not separated from the community; rather, the sisters remained at "home" in the motherhouse, where their younger peers could visit, engage, and care for them, witnessing the same peace and equanimity I witnessed during my time in the convent.

Summary: Prayer as Social Support

This chapter has examined how prayer—and, specifically, intercessions—shaped the nuns' experiences of aging. As such, this chapter brings to the fore a model of language in which language does much more than simply describe the world. The petitions functioned in the convent in multiple ways, communicating that God was available for intercession in the world and that God was present and real. By directing attention to God's presence, the prayers reminded the nuns that they were never alone. The prayers also functioned as a means of social support as the nuns communicated community needs to the divine and to each other. Finally, the prayers functioned as a mode of socialization into acceptance of decline and a celebration of death. These public prayers were a key social practice that taught the nuns to embrace aging.

4

Care, Elderspeak, and Meaningful Engagement

• •

By the time I met Sister Helen, who is pictured in figure 4.1, she had a deteriorative neurological condition that made it nearly impossible for her to speak.
She had trouble moving her hands and controlling many of her muscles. She
could communicate using the sounds "ah" and "mm," which she could vary in
rhythm and prosody. She lived in the infirmary, where nurses and her peers
bathed her, changed her clothes, took her out of bed, sat her in a chair, changed
her clothes again, and moved her back into bed at night. Each day one of the
sisters spoon-fed Sister Helen her meals.

Imagine, for a moment, interacting with Sister Helen. What would you say?
What would you be able to talk about or do together? How would you interact with someone who could not communicate with you in ways that you could
understand? In the United States, many people like Sister Helen become socially
isolated. When friends, family, or caregivers interact with people who cannot
communicate fluently, they often resort to *elderspeak,* a simplified register of
speech that resembles baby talk, the singsong manner in which many people
use to speak to infants (Grainger 1993).[1]

In the United States and western Europe, older adults who need daily care
spend much of their time alone, in an isolated environment in which they have
little social interaction (Grainger 1993). Linguist Karen Grainger has found that
even when older adults are communicatively engaged, their contributions are
often ignored or even demeaned. This bleak social landscape, with few "con-
firmative and stimulating adult-to-adult encounters," is unfortunately common

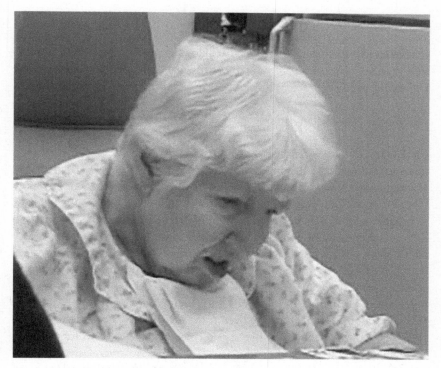

FIG. 4.1 Sister Helen. (Photo by the author)

and has been found by researchers to negatively affect elderly individuals' cognitive function (Williams 2011, 9). Grainger suggests that the "most important move" in elder care would be "for elderly long-term care to take place in an environment in which the status of caring (vs. curing) is elevated to the level of a valued occupation and skill" (1993, 433). When she wrote this, Grainger anticipated a change in aging policy by two decades. Indeed, since then, isolation and loneliness have been identified as major risk factors affecting physical and mental health in older adults (Ong, Uchino, and Wethington 2016). A number of studies have linked social isolation with shorter life spans, depression, problems in cardiovascular health, and lower reported well-being (Courtin and Knapp 2015; Ong, Uchino, and Wethington 2016). Grainger, in the quote above, suggests that instead of "curing" elders in isolation, institutions must focus on care and interaction.

Nuns offer one model of this approach, as the convent provides remarkably robust social support. To some extent Grainger's call to increase meaningful communication with older adults can be addressed by simply increasing the number of opportunities older adults have to engage with each other and with family, community members, and care providers. This, at its essence, is a matter of facilitating copresence, allowing people to be together. The one major challenge to this is the stigma attached to aging in the United States, the notion that older people in general are less capable of engaging in rich communication than are other adults. One step to reducing elderspeak in contexts with communicatively competent older adults may require a reexamination of this stigma.

Elderspeak has a handful of identifiable linguistic features, including slow speech rate, exaggerated intonation, elevated pitch and volume, simplified vocabulary, reduced grammatical complexity, changed affect, collective pronoun substitutions, diminutives, and repetition (Nussbaum et al. 1996; Ryan, Maclean, and Orange 1994; Williams 2011). A majority of older adults report that elderspeak feels patronizing and disrespectful. It has been found to result in negative self-assessment (Edwards and Noller 1993; Gould, Saum, and Belter 2002; Kemper and Harden 1999; Ryan, Hummert, and Boich 1995; Williams, Kemper, and Hummert 2003). Even more concerning, elderspeak has been linked to social isolation and cognitive decline (Salthouse 1999; Williams 2011), negative behaviors (Ryan, Maclean, and Orange 1994), and an increase in resistiveness to care (Cunningham and Williams 2007; Williams et al. 2009; Williams et al. 2016). There have been some successful interventions to train caregivers to avoid using many of the elements of elderspeak (see, for example, Williams 2013 and Williams et al. 2016). They have, however, failed to eliminate two important elements: a tendency to use simple vocabulary and reduced grammatical complexity (Corwin 2017, 2), both of which are important for maintaining cognitive and emotional well-being (Salthouse 1999; Savage, Piguet, and Hodges 2015).

Avoiding elderspeak and speaking with the same linguistic complexity and richness that individuals use with other adults should not be too difficult when individuals are interacting with communicative older adults. Yet elderspeak can be significantly harder to avoid when an older adult has linguistic difficulties that result in communicative breakdown. For instance, if an individual cannot or does not respond when he is addressed or if his responses are not clear or do not correlate with the topic of conversation, it can be difficult to engage in interaction without communicative breakdown. These breakdowns can be confusing or off-putting at the least and can be awkward, emotionally painful, or bring shame if the older adult becomes aware and/or frustrated with his inability to communicate. For instance, not being able to appropriately answer a question or collaborate in a simple two-part sequence can be challenging for both parties. Two-part sequences often require a specific type of response. For instance, the greeting "Hello" requires a type of response such as "Hello," rather than "Fourteen," and "Nice to see you" requires a particular type of answer, such as "Nice to see you, too" rather than silence or a non sequitur such as

"Window." If one of the participants is not able to participate in a culturally appropriate way, the exchange can become stressful for both interlocutors. Interacting with someone who has communicative challenges can sometimes lead caregivers or others to engage with individuals using only simplified speech or, in an effort to avoid discomfort, to begin to avoid interaction all together.

When I was in the convent, I noticed that, despite the presence of many sisters who had significant communicative difficulties, I heard almost no elderspeak. In fact, only one of the dozens of sisters I saw interacting with older sisters in the infirmary regularly used elderspeak at all. Remarkably, the sisters whom I witnessed interacting with those who had communicative difficulties engaged them using rich, linguistically complex conversations, even though the sisters could not always respond in kind. This is a remarkable achievement. Imagine, for a moment, the linguistic difficulty of this task. Most of the typical ways we interact with individuals involve mutual active and relevant participation. With the exception of reading texts or listening to monologues, communication is usually a dance in which both parties participate.

How did the nuns engage their peers who had challenges communicating in rich, linguistically complex conversations? The data for this chapter come from my time shadowing Sister Irma, Sister Rita, and other nuns who provided pastoral care to the older sisters in the infirmary. In care interactions, I found that these sisters used three linguistic strategies to engage their peers in rich interaction without speaking down to them or using elderspeak: blessings, jokes, and narratives.

Blessings

First, the visiting sister prayed. On one of the first days I followed Sister Irma room to room in the infirmary, she told me that even though she could not massage some of the sisters' feet, which was something she regularly did for most of the nuns, she always went in to check on them. I watched as she moved down the linoleum hallway, walking into each open doorway. When she encountered a sister who could not speak or move, she reached out her thumb and drew a cross on that sister's forehead and spoke a blessing, such as "Jesus told me to tell you that he loves you."

On one such visit, Sister Irma bent over the armchair Sister Jeanne was sitting in and drew the cross on the sister's head (see fig. 4.2).

Here, she spoke a blessing. As in chapter 3, the interactions are transcribed using transcription conventions that provide detail into not only *what* words were spoken but also *how* they were spoken. The conventions are explained in the appendix.

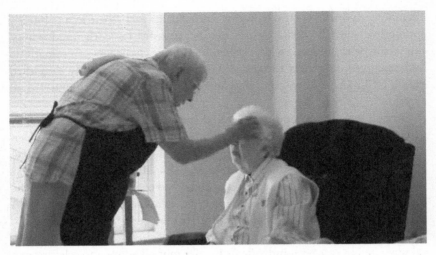

FIG. 4.2 Sister Irma drawing the sign of the cross. (Photo by the author)

EXAMPLE 1: BLESSING

```
01      May the Lord bless you
02      and keep you
03      and give you peace
04      in your heart.
```

Although the blessing was short, it nevertheless demonstrates relative grammatical complexity, with multiple clauses that engaged Sister Jeanne without requiring her to respond. Because blessings are structured such that the direct recipient is the divine and not the human subject of the prayer, the interaction would be communicatively "successful" whether or not Sister Jeanne responded.

While Sister Jeanne had the opportunity to be engaged in meaningful interaction, she was not required to respond in a particular way. Thus, whether she was silent or responded, she could be a "successful" participant in a rich and meaningful interaction.

Sister Irma often requested blessings from the older sisters in the infirmary, including those who had limited communicative ability. For instance, in the following exchange, Sister Irma walked into Sister Helen's room. Sister Helen, whom we met at the beginning of this chapter, had a deteriorative neurological disorder which limited her ability to speak clearly. She seemed to understand language when she was spoken to and she could produce a few sounds such as "ah" and "mm" with some variation in prosody by increasing and decreasing the pitch contours and rhythm of these sounds. It was extremely difficult to make out what she was trying to say, which made communication challenging.

After Sister Irma massaged Sister Helen's feet and washed her hands, she asked Sister Helen if she would like a blessing. Sister Helen responded with "mm." As we saw in the exchange above, the blessing afforded a rich linguistic exchange even if the recipient could not produce clear words. After her blessing, Sister Irma asked Sister Helen to bless her in return. As I sat on Sister Helen's bed, holding my audio recorder, I remember being a bit stunned by this request. How could she ask someone who could produce only a variation of moans to provide a blessing for her?

I watched as Sister Irma placed Sister Helen's hand on her forehead and listened while Sister Helen blessed her:

EXAMPLE 2: SISTER HELEN'S BLESSING

Participants

SI: Sister Irma
SH: Sister Helen
AC: Anna Corwin (author)

01 SI: There ya go::
02   (6.0)
03   You ready for your blessing?
04 SH: Ahhhhhsh.
05 SI: Okay.
06   (5.0)
07   May the Lord bless you and keep you. May He give
08   you courage to live each day knowing He is with
09   you.
10   Amen.
11   (1.5)
12 SH: Ahhh.
13 SI: And now I'd like to have a blessing, okay?
14   Can you bless me?
15 SH: Mmmhhh, mmhh, mmhhh, mmhh, mmmhhh,
16   mmmhh ahhh.
17   Mhh mm-hmm, mmmmm, mm-mm.
18 SI: Amen. Thank you.
19 SH: Ahh.

After the blessing was completed, Sister Irma invited Sister Helen to give me a blessing. She called me over and placed Sister Helen's hand on my forehead (line 22).

20 SI: Would you like to give Anna a blessing too?
21 AC: I would love that if—

```
22 SI:   C'mon over this side.
23 AC:   Thank you Sister.
24 SH:   Ahhhhh. MMMMmmmmmm. Mmmmmmm. Mmmmmmmmmm.
25 AC:   Amen.
26 SH:   AAhhmmmm.
27 AC:   Thank you, Sister; thank you so much.
28 SH:   Aaahhh.
29 SI:   She's still blessing.
30 SH:   Aaahh, ahhh, ahhhh, mmhhh.
31 SI:   (. . .)
32 AC:   Bless you, Sister.
33       ((Running water))
34 SH:   Mmmhhh, mmhh.
35 SI:   (. . .)
36 SH:   Mmhhh, mmhh, mmmhhh, mmmhh.
```

Being a non-Catholic and not skilled in receiving blessings, I thanked Sister Helen (line 27) before she had finished. She ignored my blunder and kept going, and Sister Irma kindly explained to me that she was still in the middle of the blessing (line 29).

Even though Sister Helen was the one who could use only a few sounds and variation in prosody to communicate, it was me, the non-Catholic, who was the only incompetent participant. As was typical in my first few months at the convent, I had not yet learned the patterns of prayer well enough to participate fluently, and as usual, the nuns gracefully alerted me to my errors and helped me learn.

Despite her limited communicative ability Sister Helen, unlike me, was able to be a competent participant in the blessing, not only as Sister Irma engaged her in dynamic interaction but also as she produced her own prayers. The fact that Sister Irma and I could not understand the prayer did not matter for the communicative success of the interaction, since the primary recipient was God. Blessings, therefore, allowed for individuals like Sister Helen to participate as both a listener and a speaker in linguistically rich, meaningful interaction free of the trappings of elderspeak.

Jokes

Sister Irma had a remarkable array of jokes. There was the one about the donkey on whom Jesus rode into Jerusalem who, upon hearing the cries of the people—"Hosanna! Blessed is he who comes in the name of the Lord!"—trotted a little bit more proudly, thinking to himself, "My name must be Hosanna!" And there was the one about the old couple who sat in the kitchen, and one morning the man asked the woman "Honey, do I wear boxers or briefs?"

and she answered, "Depends." No matter how many times I heard her jokes, Irma's impish smile and chuckles always filled me with a lightness and joy.

Dementia can be terrifying as it renders familiar landscapes unfamiliar and steals memories and familiar faces. It can take the humdrum of quotidian conversation and create a minefield from it. One morning, as I walked the hallways after Mass, I saw Sister Julette walking toward me. Sister Julette was one of the few sisters who still wore a habit with a veil. I stopped to make small talk and asked her if she had enjoyed the Mass. The muscles in her face went slack and a look of fear, if not terror, washed over her. Had Mass already happened? She was heading there and could not remember if she had already been or if she had overslept and forgotten. As I tried to reassure her that it was okay, Sister Julette became increasingly lost in a confusion and a moral panic that she had done something wrong by (unintentionally) skipping Mass. Another sister soon saw us in the hallway and with a much more forceful authority reassured Sister Julette that everything was all right.

This moment, as my seemingly mild small talk created such suffering in a woman who could no longer rely on her sense of time and memory to get herself to Mass, brought home to me how devastating dementia can be. The routine stability of time and space and the familiarity of the world could become corrupted and confused. This story ended well enough—the sisters quickly coordinated efforts so that in the future Sister Julette always had someone come by to accompany her to Mass—but it made me aware that even routine daily communication like the small talk I tried to engage in with Sister Julette could become quite difficult for people experiencing dementia and other pronounced cognitive decline.

In the following interaction, Sister Irma, who had known Sister Julette for most of their lives, entered Sister Julette's room to provide a foot massage. Sister Julette began the exchange by remarking that she had forgotten Sister Irma's name. The fact that she said "and I forgot" indicates that she was aware that she had once known and perhaps *should* have known Sister Irma's name. This was a potentially delicate exchange as it brought to the fore the fact that Sister Julette was rapidly losing her memory, but Sister Irma skillfully transitioned to joking.

EXAMPLE 3: JOKING
Participants
```
SI:    Sister Irma
SJ:    Sister Julette

01 SJ:  And I forgot your name.
02 SI:  Irma.
03 SJ:  Irma.
04 SI:  We used to play cards together.
05 SJ:  Irma . . . ?
```

```
06 SI:   Coleman.
07 SJ:   Coleman.
08 SI:   Sister Irma. Sometimes some of 'em call me Fatty
09       Irma,
10       or Ratty Irma, or Bratty Irma.
11       I get all kinds. But then I give 'em right back.
12       (heh. heh. hheeh)
13 SJ:   You don't pay attention to any of 'em.
14 SI:   Nah, it's fun. They're just teasing me. Right?
15       You learn how to take a teasing.
```

The joking that Sister Irma used here moved the conversation away from the potentially upsetting reminder that Sister Julette had forgotten the name of someone she had known for decades. It also allowed the two nuns to communicate using linguistically rich and complex language (Corwin 2018). In addition, the joking allowed Sister Julette to join in the interaction while not requiring her to contribute in a specific way.

In this exchange, Sister Julette participated by joining Sister Irma in laughter (line 12) and through speech (line 13), but her participation was not required for the interaction to unfold coherently. This is an important feature of joking, a genre of speech that allows participants the opportunity to engage linguistically, but even if they say nothing, or only smile or chuckle, participants such as Sister Julette would be included in a linguistically rich communicative interaction.

Narratives

Another strategy that the sisters used in the infirmary was the recounting of narratives. This strategy was similar to joking in that it allowed the sisters to engage in rich, linguistically complex interaction with other sisters who might not have been able to respond to other types of communication. Narratives allowed rich and varied engagement without requiring a specific response from an interlocutor. They did, however, allow the communicative partner to engage in a subsequent story if she chose to. In this way, much like blessings and jokes, narratives allowed for linguistic engagement with people who had limited communicative ability while simultaneously providing a very low risk of communicative breakdown.

In the following example, which occurred a few minutes after the joke mentioned above, Sister Irma was massaging Sister Julette's feet. She raised a potentially problematic topic, the recent death of a mutual friend, a peer in the convent whom Sister Julette had known well but might have forgotten. In this interaction, we can see that the question-and-answer formulation at the beginning (lines 01–04) was problematic, as Sister Julette had forgotten that her friend Sister Alice had died. Sister Irma responded to the tension created in this question-and-answer sequence by beginning a narrative.

EXAMPLE 4: NARRATIVES
Participants
SI: Sister Irma
SJ: Sister Julette
AC: Anna Corwin (author)

```
01 SI:   Did you know sister Alice?
02 SJ:   Oh yes.
03 SI:   You know she died?
04 SJ:   Oh?
05 SI:   Yeah, she died very suddenly.
06       So we had her prayer service today in,
07       down in the, memorial service.
08       And they told funny stories about her.
09 SJ:   Oh.
10 SI:   One night the lights went out where they lived.
11       And, they always played cards at night.
12       But she would never,
13       she didn't want to play cards.
14       She'd never play.
15       That night, they had candles around.
16       So,
17       she came out with 'em 'cause she didn't want to be
18       in the dark.
19       And she played and she won!
20       She won the game (heh.h.hah) and enjoyed it!
21       I thought that was=
22 AC:   =That was wonderful.
23 SJ:   Yeah, she's a nice person.
24 SI:   Yes. She ended up being a librarian.
```

The narrative not only resolved the social tension that was introduced in the question-and-answer sequence (in lines 01–04) but also allowed Sister Irma to communicate using linguistically complex language without requiring Sister Julette to say anything specific. Sister Julette did not have to affirm or deny any particular memories and could successfully participate in the interaction whether or not she remembered or could produce specific memories or language. The structure of the narrative allowed her to participate if she chose to, as she did in line 23, "Yes, she's a nice person," but the interaction would also have been communicatively successful without her participation. In this way, narratives, like blessings and jokes, allowed the sisters to interact with their peers who had communicative limits using meaningful, linguistically rich and grammatically complex language.

Social Engagement: Playing Cards Together

The nuns not only engaged each other in complex linguistic interactions while they provided structured care, as Sister Irma did in the instances above, but also in meaningful social interactions whose purpose was not explicitly to provide care. For instance, Sister Helen, whom Sister Irma had asked to pray for me despite her productive aphasia, was fed, dressed, bathed, and physically cared for; but she was also engaged as a meaningful participant in everyday social activities. Almost every evening, after the sisters had finished supper, two nuns, Sister Polly and Sister Marie, would play cards with Sister Helen.

The idea that Sister Helen, with limited ability to express herself verbally and move physically, would be able to engage in a card game might seem far-fetched. One might picture, for instance, a game in which Sisters Polly and Marie *played at* playing cards with Sister Helen to humor her or express care for her. One could imagine a unidirectional activity in which Sister Helen's peers played with her to amuse or edify her, but this was not what happened. The card game was not an activity set up to care *for* Sister Helen. This was an honest and remarkably competitive game in which all three women were engaged in a meaningful activity together.

Before we turn to examine *how* Sisters Polly and Marie engaged Sister Helen in a meaningful game of cards, it is important to note *that* they engaged her in this activity in the first place. This is further evidence of the pattern in the convent in which individuals were valued even after they were no longer active or productive adults. Although Sister Helen's physical and communicative abilities were limited, her peers continued to treat her as a valuable member of the community. Rather than being segregated from the ongoing activities in the convent, Sister Helen continued to be invited to participate in social activities such as the lively card games that many of the sisters played each night. This is evidence of the ideology in the convent that all persons were valuable and meaningful members of the community. Echoing chapter 2, this is another example of how, through their everyday interactions, the sisters communicated to each other the idea that every person was valuable at every stage of the life course. By publicly engaging sisters like Sister Helen in meaningful social activities, they were communicating to each other and to younger peers the community expectations about aging and engagement across the life course.

Beyond noting that community members engaged peers like Sister Helen in this way, one must ask *how* the two sisters played a meaningful and relatively competitive game of cards with Sister Helen. The exchange that follows provides a glimpse into their interactions. What is remarkable about the way in which they engage with Sister Helen is that the sisters provided just enough scaffolding to allow Sister Helen to maximize her participation, allowing her to participate to the maximum of her ability.[2]

EXAMPLE 5: PLAYING CARDS
Participants
SM: Sister Marie
SH: Sister Helen
SP: Sister Polly

The three have been playing cards for five minutes
at the start of this transcript.

```
01 SM:  Eight, nine, ten.
02      This needs an eleven.
03      Six, seven, eight; this needs a nine.
04      Needs a nine. Needs eleven.
05 SP:  (. . .)
06 SM:  ((Pulls card from deck, places it on table in front
07      of SH))
08      Helen, have you got a ni:ne?
09      Or a five or a two?
10      Or an eleven?
11      You've got an eleven down there ((pointing)).
12      ((Pulls card from deck, places it on table in front
13      of SH))
14 SH:  ((Pulls card from hand, places it on the table))
15 SM:  Have you got a nine?
16 SP:  You can play your two over here.
17      ((SM and SP both touch cards on the table in front
18      of SH))
19 SM:  ((Flips over a card that is in front of SH))
20 SM:  ((Pulls card from deck, places it in front of SH's
21      body))
22 SH:  ((Takes the card from SM))
23 SM:  Now you need a—
24 SH:  ((Moves card from hand onto table))
25 SM:  ((Takes card from SH and puts it on pile in the
```

```
26        middle of the table))
27        Now you need a—a ten. You've got a ten here.
28        ((Pointing))
29 SH:    ((Reaches for card from a pile on the table))
30 SM:    ((Puts her hand on the pile, and this prevents SH
31        from taking a card))
32        Nope, that's a four.
33        That won't play, Helen.
34        Your ten will play ((touching cards)).
35        Your ten and your eleven and your two will all play.
36 SH:    ((Moves card from hand to table))
37 SM:    ((Takes card from SH and puts it on pile in the
38        middle of the table))
39 SM:    Eleven.
40 SM:    ((Takes card from SH and puts it on pile in the
41        middle of the table))
```

In the first five lines of the transcript Sister Marie provided just enough verbal context to allow Sister Helen to engage by listing the cards aloud. When Sister Helen did not make a move, Sister Marie asked her explicitly if she had the card that was needed (line 08). When Sister Helen did not respond, she provided even more direct scaffolding, pointing out that Sister Helen had a card that would play (line 11). She then pulled another card from the deck and placed it in front of Sister Helen. During this sequence, Sister Helen was relatively still and remained slumped over, with her hands under the table. It was not immediately apparent to me that she was listening or attending to the ongoing game. An uninformed viewer of the video recording might have mistaken her for someone who was sleeping. Then, for anyone watching who did not know Sister Helen, something remarkable happened. In line 14, Sister Helen's hand slowly emerges from under the table and she places a card from her hand on the table demonstrating that she was not only attending to the game but was engaged as an active participant.

In the following lines, Sisters Polly and Marie continued to provide just enough scaffolding to allow Sister Helen to participate without going so far as to do things for her or to limit her possible actions in any way. In each moment, her peers allowed Sister Helen to maximize her participation before providing assistance. In line 29, when Sister Helen reached for a card that would not "play" with the cards that were out, instead of making a play for her, Sister Marie simply placed her hand over the pile Sister Helen was moving her hand toward. This allowed Sister Helen to correct course on her own. A moment later, Sister Helen reached out to place a card on a pile on the table but could not reach the

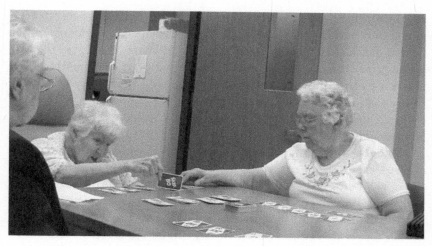

FIG. 4.3 Sister Helen reaches out to place a card on a pile on the table. (Photo by the author)

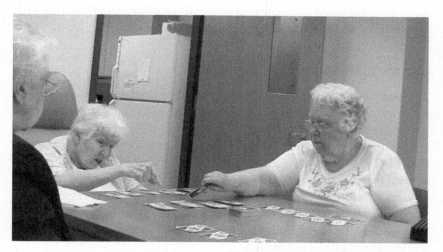

FIG. 4.4 When Sister Helen has maximized her reach, Sister Marie completes the action. (Photo by the author)

full distance (see fig. 4.3). Just at the moment when Sister Helen had maximized her reach, extending her arm with the card, Sister Marie seamlessly took hold of the card and continued the flow of action, placing it on the pile Sister Helen had been moving it toward (see fig. 4.4).

Watching Sisters Marie, Polly, and Helen play cards together felt to me like watching a well-choreographed dance. Sister Helen was included as a meaningful participant, and the other sisters were present to assist her when she came to the edge of her physical capacity. The sisters never stepped in too soon, which would have limited Sister Helen's full participation, but neither did they leave her hanging, which would have interrupted the flow of the game. Sister Helen moved slowly, but her peers consistently waited until she had maximized her action before stepping in, and they were attentive enough that when she reached the edge of her possible participation, they were there to finish the action or provide scaffolding to allow for a subsequent action.

Much like the blessings, jokes, and narratives that Sister Irma and others engaged in with their peers, social interactions like this card game allowed for sisters who were experiencing age-related decline to participate meaningfully in dynamic social interaction. Notably, these interactions were not unidirectional activities in which a caregiver attended to someone who could no longer care for herself. Instead, these activities were meaningful joint activities in which peers engaged each other. By continuing to engage sisters like Sister Julette and Sister Helen in social activities, the community provided opportunities for aging sisters to be engaged physically and linguistically to the maximum of their ability in meaningful cooperative activities.

Summary: Meaningful Engagement

The linguistic techniques that the nuns used in the convent offered opportunities for each sister to listen and produce meaningful interaction and to be engaged in lexically and grammatically rich conversation without pressure to engage in ways that were beyond her ability and without risking failure. The sisters skillfully engaged their peers with blessings, jokes, and narratives that allowed them to engage meaningfully even when their peers could not respond in kind. In addition, as we saw with Sister Helen's card game, they also provided opportunities for sisters to maximize their possible participation, to continue to engage meaningfully, and therefore not risk atrophy of their social and linguistic abilities or isolation.

Given how detrimental elderspeak can be for individuals' physical and emotional health, these examples illustrate important alternatives. The sisters' communicative strategies not only avoided elderspeak but engaged communicatively compromised older adults as respected peers, exposing them to linguistically complex, grammatically rich interaction that has been documented to help maintain emotional and cognitive health.

This concludes part I of the book, which has focused on the ways in which the nuns' ideologies and practices fit into the "successful aging" paradigm—a paradigm I have critiqued for its antiaging assumptions. In part II we will look at how the nuns' practices and ideologies have changed over the sisters' lifetimes. As we will see in the chapters 5–7, the major institutional changes that occurred in the Catholic Church following Vatican II have had significant impacts on the nuns' lives and therefore on their linguistic practices and their experiences in the world. Chapter 5 examines how prayer practices drastically changed between the time nuns entered the convent and the time I arrived; the chapter will look at how the changes in the structure of prayer shaped how the nuns experienced their own bodies, illness, and pain. Chapter 6 will then look at how ideologies of pain have changed over the same time period, and chapter 7 will look at how Vatican II shaped some of the nuns' theological practices, including the meaning of their vows and their relationship with self-determination and material goods. This, too, had implications for how the nuns experienced aging.

Together the chapters in part II look to the institutional event that changed the course of the nuns' lives, Vatican II, detailing how their habitual practices were reshaped. We will begin to see how the transformation has led to a particular moment in time in which we see the nuns and their attitudes about and experiences of aging. We will see that cultural practices are not fixed but always in contact with the ever-changing political, historical, and social structures in the world.

Part 2

Shaping Experience

•••••••••••••••••••••••

The Convent in
Sociohistorical Context

5

Changing God, Changing Bodies

● ●

How Prayer Practices Shape
Embodied Experience

When I met Sister Theresa she was eighty-three years old. She had a soft round face and a tremendous laugh. When she was seventeen years old, in 1944, Sister Theresa left a large German Catholic family in the rural Midwest to join the Franciscan Sisters of the Sacred Heart Convent. After becoming a nun, she spent decades teaching and working as a missionary. In the 1960s she was one of the first five sisters from the convent to travel to Oceania to work as a missionary. See figure 5.1 for an image of S. Theresa leaving for her mission work. While in Oceania, she developed amebiasis, a parasitic infection of amoebas that spread throughout her body. The condition went untreated for years, and by the time she returned to the United States in the early 1970s her infection was incurable. For more than thirty years, Sister Theresa had trouble walking as a result of the amebiasis. She retired early and spent the rest of her life living in the convent. By the end of her life, her movement was limited. With significant effort, she could walk only a few steps; she used a motorized wheelchair to move through the convent. She had had a number of surgeries to remove infected areas of her body, and in 2009, portions of her feet had to be amputated due to the amebiasis.

Sitting in a plush easy chair in her small room in the assisted living wing of the convent, Sister Theresa told me that for years she interpreted the pain as

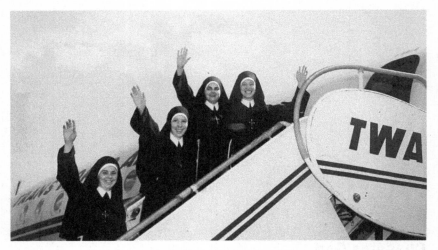

FIG. 5.1 Sister Theresa and peers leaving for Oceania. (Photo courtesy of the archives of the Sisters of the Sacred Heart Convent)

God's will and she used to ask God why she had had to endure such physical and mental suffering. She used to curse the amoebas infecting her body and pray that God would heal her. What occurred next in Sister Theresa's narrative was afforded by changes in convent prayer life following Vatican II, and the ideological shift that accompanied these changes. She said that a few decades before I met her, while she was praying, she realized that "if everything in the world is divine," as she had been taught in the convent after Vatican II, "if every single creature is not only made by God but *is* God" then it seemed only logical that the amoebas infecting her body must be God as well. Upon realizing this, she said, "I called a meeting of all the amoebas in my body and apologized." She spoke to them, saying "the same creator made us all." She said that now she loved "her" amoebas as she loved God, and every morning she would stand in front of the mirror and address all of God within herself, including the amoebas, in her daily prayer. She said that although she still experienced pain, this pain was no longer as significant as it once was. She no longer interpreted her pain as divine punishment. Sister Theresa told me that when she let go of the idea of divine punishment and began to interpret the pain as a natural part of God's world, the level of her pain decreased.

This radical shift in Sister Theresa's thinking and in the trajectory of her chronic pain experience was shaped by the institutional changes implemented in the convent during the twentieth century. Like the majority of her peers, prior to the institutional change in the Church associated with Vatican II, Sister Theresa saw God as an authority responsible for her suffering, a figure to whom she addressed her problems and concerns about her illness. After Vatican II, she came to see God as so thoroughly integrated into every creature on earth that she came to address the amoebas infecting her body as part of a loving God. Through this process, Sister Theresa's concept of her body was transformed such that she began to experience the divine within the bounds of her physical body, even in the amoebic cells infecting her. Her *epistemology of pain*, her understanding of what pain is, changed as she stopped associating her pain with divine punishment and began interpreting it as an index of the oneness of God with the world. Sister Theresa's narrative exemplifies contemporary arguments that the experience of pain is deeply tied to cultural and individual interpretations of illness and pain. Or, as David Morris has articulated, "pain is experienced only as it is interpreted" (1991, 29).

This chapter looks at the historical shift in institutional prayer practices in the church.[1] While at first Vatican II may not appear to be connected to the sisters' health outcomes, Sister Theresa's story gives us a glimpse into how a historical shift in the Church impacted the nuns' experiences of their bodies. As Sister Theresa changed the way she addressed God, a transformation inspired by institutional changes that began in Rome, five thousand miles away, she also felt changes in how pain manifested in her body. The ethnography of this institutional transformation affords insight into the ways the nuns experience aging and well-being.

In this chapter, I explore the institutional and personal transformations that afforded a profound linguistic and embodied shift as nuns like Sister Theresa began to address God as a divine being within their bodies instead of as an authority outside or above them. I explore how these transformations altered the nuns' cultural and moral interpretation of pain as they began to experience chronic illness as a sense of unity with the divine instead of pain and suffering delivered by God. I rely on linguistic analysis of the nuns' narratives to show how their prayer practices were central in changing their *somatic modes of attention*, the processes through which they attend to and experience their bodies and the embodied presence of others (Csordas 1993).

How people experience pain is an important aspect of the aging process. As individuals age, they can experience more chronic pain as the body makes itself known in new ways. How one experiences this pain is connected to how one understands and experiences aging and what it means to grow older in the world.

God before Vatican II

For centuries, in convents across the world, Catholic nuns were taught to pray on schedule, rising before dawn to meet God in language that they had memorized as young novices. Nuns were trained to silently recite memorized prayers even as they completed each of their daily tasks. As the Franciscan Sisters of

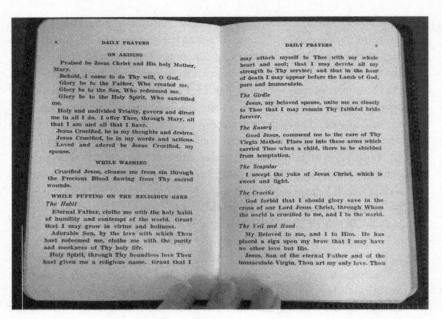

FIG. 5.2 A daily prayer book. (Photo by the author)

the Sacred Heart descended the convent steps in their woolen habits to begin work each day in the sweltering summer humidity and in the frigid January cold, they were to recite, "Meek and humble Jesus, who didst descend to the lowliness of the tomb, grant that I may always descend below all creatures by practicing true humility."

These prayers, memorized from the community's prayer manual, inscribed every act, from washing and eating to moving through the convent. A photograph of the prayer manual appears in figure 5.2. When they bathed the nuns spoke the words "Crucified Jesus, cleanse me from sin through Thy Precious Blood flowing from Thy sacred wounds." When they dressed, they spoke a silent prayer for each piece of the habit as they put it on. Tying on the girdle, they prayed, "Jesus, unite me as closely to Thee that I may remain Thy faithful bride forever." Just as the details of their days—from what they ate to where they worked—were shaped by the Church authorities, the nuns' private conversations with the divine were scripted and their relationship with the divine was thus sculpted by the Church.

In the 1960s, all of this changed. In 1959, when Pope John XXIII convened the Second Ecumenical Council of the Vatican, or Vatican II, a meeting of Church authorities, he set out to "renew" the Catholic Church and to promote "unity and grace" across Catholic communities worldwide (O'Malley 2008). For many Catholics, including the Franciscan Sisters of the Sacred Heart,

Vatican II seemed to break open the Church, letting in flexibility and the freedom to work and pray as they chose.

Joan Chittister, a Benedictine nun, has written that nuns experienced far greater institutional change than anyone else in the Church. She describes the lives of nuns in the years following Vatican II as a "maelstrom of massive social change" and "the vortex of an institutional storm" at "ground zero of organizational meltdown" (2003, 23). Although the majority of the nuns in the Franciscan Sisters of the Sacred Heart Convent describe the changes following Vatican II in a positive light, Chittister's description provides insight into the scale of the change as it affected the lives of nuns, as well as the speed of its implementation. One sister in my study who had left the community for ten years and rejoined following Vatican II told me that when she reentered, she was shocked by the scope and scale of the changes in the convent during that decade. She called the scale of the changes in the convent "phenomenal."

Only one document that was issued from Rome dealt directly with the changes to be effected in monasteries and convents. Given the significance of the changes that were made in religious life, the document is surprisingly brief. In *Decree on the Adaptation and Renewal of Religious Life: Perfectae Caritatis*, the Vatican Council declared that, in convents, "The manner of living, praying and working should be suitably adapted everywhere . . . as required by the nature of each institute, to the necessities of the apostolate, the demands of culture, and social and economic circumstances. Therefore let constitutions, directories, custom books, books of prayers and ceremonies and such like be suitably re-edited and, obsolete laws being suppressed, be adapted to the decrees of this sacred synod" (Vatican Council 1965). The decree emphasized a return to the charism or inspiration of each community, giving each convent the power to decide which changes would be appropriate to make. So while Vatican II commanded extensive changes, it did not dictate these changes in detail, and sisters in each religious community were allowed to modify their convents' practices as they saw fit according to the history and values of that community. This resulted in a great diversity of practices in modern convent life. Some convents saw no change, while many, like the Franciscan Sisters of the Sacred Heart Convent, saw significant transformations in virtually all aspects of the sisters' lives. Since the changes following Vatican II were so slowly instituted, many of the sisters who lived through them have said that it was not until many years after Vatican II that they realized the scale of the changes that had occurred. In the thirty-one life history interviews I conducted in the convent, Vatican II was rarely described. In narratives, it was constructed as a hinge— both binding and acting as a divider between the time periods that straddle it. These narratives illustrate Mary Jo Weaver's claim that "American Catholicism in the twentieth century divides neatly down the middle" (1999, 154).

Along with a progressive elimination of the habit worn by the nuns, the restructuring of the nuns' daily schedules, and changes in authority structure and in the concept of obedience, Vatican II also brought about a significant shift in almost all of the linguistic practices in which the sisters participated. Liturgy, which had been spoken in Latin, was now spoken in English. Prayer books were edited to accommodate a new intimacy with the divine and to be more inclusive of all people. Daily prayers transitioned from highly structured and scripted forms to free, individually designed forms of communion with God. Before Vatican II, the sisters were required to follow a uniform schedule, praying from set texts at set times throughout the day. After Vatican II, they were encouraged to set their own daily schedules and pray however and whenever they chose. For the sisters who still worked, this meant that they had more flexibility in scheduling their prayer life around their responsibilities. The changes following Vatican II also included an elimination of rules restricting the sisters' interactions with each other. Rules forbidding social interaction and conversational exchanges were abandoned, allowing the sisters to cultivate closer relationships with each other in the convent. Finally, the convent moved from a hierarchical structure of authority to a more democratic model of shared responsibility (Ruether 1991).

In addition to these changes, the nuns were affected by ideological changes embraced by the Church after Vatican II, including the resignification of pain and suffering. The Franciscan Sisters of the Sacred Heart described a dual notion of pain similar to that described by Robert Orsi in his writing about Catholics' sense of suffering in the early twentieth century. Pain was understood to have the character of a sacrament, helping one achieve closeness with the divine, and simultaneously was interpreted as an act of punishment sent down from the divine (Orsi 2005, 22–23). These ideologies changed in the decades following Vatican II. The nuns spoke of a time when they had "mistakenly" understood pain to be punishment sent down from God in response to human sin. They said that after Vatican II they "understood" that God did not cause pain and suffering; rather, he was a companion helping them endure it. While they used to accept pain as "God's will" for them and pray for him to change his "will" and take away the pain, their new prayers focused on acceptance and communion with the divine in the face of pain. Chapter 6 will explore in greater detail this history of pain in the Church and its role in the sisters' notions of healing.

This change comprises a major shift in the concept of *divine agency* in human suffering, away from concepts of God as the arbiter of pain to that of a companion who can help the sisters endure pain. Many of the sisters said that they felt they were "no longer alone" in their pain, and, like Sister Theresa, a number of them reported that this feeling of companionship helped to lessen the impact of their chronic pain.

Prayer and the Body

As we saw in chapter 4, the Franciscan Sisters of the Sacred Heart pray to fulfill a number of practical and ideological goals. They pray to connect to the
divine, to strengthen communal bonds, to better themselves, to "purify" the
body and soul (Lester 2005; Norris 2009), and to ask the divine to intercede
in worldly affairs. As a daily ritual practice, prayer organizes their days; it is a
means for spiritual growth, and it has a significant role in representing and shaping the moral and ideological world of the convent. In this chapter, I focus on
prayer as a ritual practice in which the nuns connect with the divine through
linguistic and embodied modalities: how prayer impacts the nuns' experiences
of their bodies.

As we saw in chapter 3, prayer can be a two-party or multiparty interaction
between the divine and one or more individuals through which individuals try
to "creat[e] an encounter" with the divine, who is a subjectively experienced yet
invisible presence (Hanks 1996, 171; see also James 1982; and Keane 1997). Prayer
is therefore designed not only to communicate with a divine interlocutor but
also to facilitate an *experience* of the divine (Capps and Ochs 2002; Ferguson
1985; Hanks 1996). It is through the remarkable power of language that individuals render an invisible interlocutor subjectively real. Prayer, therefore, makes
the divine both publicly and subjectively accessible.

Communication with the divine is not exclusively verbal but also *embodied*, involving the body on a number of levels. There are three ways in which
prayer involves the body: first, as a semiotic resource, or set of signs, to communicate with the divine and other congregants; second, as an object of prayer;
and, third, as embodied intersubjective interaction with the divine.

The Body as a Semiotic Resource

In prayer the body is used as a set of signs, or as a *semiotic resource* to communicate with the divine (see Capps and Ochs 2002). When entering a Catholic
church, for example, congregants kneel, bow to the altar, and inscribe the sign of
the cross over their body—bringing the fingers of one hand from the forehead
to the breast, and then from the left shoulder to the right to signify the cross and
Jesus's suffering—to communicate humility and reverence toward the divine.
These practices and other similar embodied practices across religious contexts
are linked to particular ideologies such as order, discipline, or moral selfhood
(Simon 2009; Starrett 1995; Yafeh 2007). Although this is an important aspect
of prayer, I do not analyze this aspect of embodiment directly in this chapter.

The Body as an Object of Prayer

The body is implicated as an object in many types of healing and intercessory
prayers. For example, when individuals pray for healing through a laying on of

hands (Csordas 1994, 2008), incanting God's name (Dein 2002), or petitioning for intercession, the divine is called to act on a patient's body, thus making
the body the material object of prayer. Sister Theresa exemplified this relationship between prayer and the body when she prayed to the divine to heal her
from the amoebas infecting her body.

Embodied Prayer

Finally, the body is involved directly in prayer as individuals experience a divine
presence. Thomas Csordas (1994) describes how individuals come to experience
the divine through various *sensory modalities*, and Tanya Luhrmann explores
how individuals learn to attend to their experience and understand it as evidence of the divine (Luhrmann 2005; Luhrmann, Nusbaum, and Thisted 2010).
Many of the nuns described prayer as an experience of communion with God
in which the divine was experienced through somatic, or corporeal, modalities. Some of the sisters described the experience of holding Jesus's hand, of
engaging in a divine embrace in which they felt his arms around them, or of
experiencing the divine as a calming or loving presence in the room with them.

All three of these modalities were central to the nuns' prayer practices. As
the sisters prayed they attended to the body as a resource they could use to communicate to the divine, as an object to be acted upon by the divine, and as a
resource through which they experienced the divine.

Luhrmann (2005) argues that this process of recognizing the embodied
presence of the divine requires repeated practice. Luhrmann, Nusbaum, and
Thisted show that through the repetitive practice of prayer, people "acquire the
cognitive and linguistic patterns that helped them to identify God's presence."
Through this learning process, they argue that individuals "come to see differently, to think differently, and above all to feel differently" (2010, 67–68). I will
suggest that this prayer practice can impact not only how individuals learn to
think and feel, as Luhrmann outlines, but also how they embody experiences
of illness and pain. Crucial to this relationship between prayer and the body is
a phenomenological understanding of the body in which the body is analyzed
within the context of lived experience. So framed, chronic pain and illness are
understood not to be an "external attack on our biochemical organism, but
rather a subjectively profound . . . variation in our embodiment" (Turner
1997, 17). Work in psychological and medical anthropology over the past two
decades has shown that bodily experiences such as pain are social and are
influenced by "meanings, relationships, and institutions" (Kleinman et al.
1994, 7). Central to this argument is that the way people conceive of pain is
shaped by both culture and their experiences in the world.

Although the connection between the experience of pain and sociocultural
factors shaping its interpretation has been well established, work has only begun
to untangle the process through which this occurs. Rebecca Seligman, for

example, has argued that changing patterns of attention are central to Brazilian Candomblé healing. In her work, Seligman describes an embodied process in which individuals engaging in Candomblé trance healing practices transform their patterns of attention and behavior using embodied cultural and spiritual practices to "deconstruct" and "repair" the self in ways that ameliorate distress and physical suffering (2010, 314). She argues that psychophysiological and embodied mechanisms of Candomblé healing are central to the participants' successful alleviation of physical distress and pain.

The various ways we experience our bodies and illness come to us through culturally meaningful learned processes. Cognitive psychologist Lawrence Barsalou and his colleagues argue that the states associated with religious experiences are achieved through embodied ritual. He suggests that performing embodied rituals such as taking communion "help drive people's cognitive systems into appropriate religious states" and that these embodiments "help entrench religious ideas in memory" (Barsalou et al. 2005, 49). They argue that experience is shaped by repetition of embodied acts and that specific acts influence an individual's experience. For example, they posit that the embodied acts of bowing or stilling the body in meditation aid in creating the subjective experiences of humility or mental stillness. These studies support my claim that the embodied metaphors that Catholic nuns cultivate during prayer impact their experience of the world. In a learning process similar to that described by Seligman, embodied religious ritual enables the alleviation of chronic pain.

When the Franciscan Sisters of the Sacred Heart prayed, they directed their attention to a divine interlocutor. This was an embodied process in all three ways outlined above: they used their bodies to pray (assuming a particular position on the pew and using symbols such as the sign of the cross); they sometimes prayed about their and other bodies; and they experienced divine presence through their bodies. The process through which the nuns directed their attention to the embodied presence of the divine was a fundamentally linguistic process. It was through the language of prayer that they begin to experience the divine. As Elinor Ochs argues, linguistic enactments are experienced as they are produced and perceived (2012, 5). In other words, as the nuns used language to speak to God in particular ways, they created and embodied particular experiences. As they prayed, they were experiencing the utterances that they were producing and hearing. This practice, repeated for them many times each day, impacted the ways in which they experienced their bodies and the world. In Ochs's words, "perfectly ordinary enactments of language in everyday life" become crucial "experiential moments" in individuals' lives (2012, 7). In this way, it is the language the nuns use to communicate with the divine that shapes their embodied experience as they pray.

The language we use each day produces our everyday experiences. When the language of the nuns' prayers changed following Vatican II, experience in the world shifted with it as they spoke new words. The nuns' relationship with the divine, their embodied experience of the divine, and their experience of their own bodies, including illness and pain, were profoundly transformed.

Prayer in the Convent

The convent authorities scheduled a number of activities throughout the week in which the retired sisters could participate; these included spiritual development programs, lectures, prayer meetings, exercise classes, and social activities. In the summer of 2009 the sisters in the convent adopted a new prayer book, or breviary. For the previous two decades they had been using a book published by Carmelite nuns, but the then recent release of a Franciscan breviary motivated a convent-wide change. As part of this institutional transition, a local priest was invited to give a lecture about the new prayer book to the sisters living in the assisted living and infirmary wings of the convent.

At 3:00 p.m. on a humid summer afternoon, nearly thirty of the elderly sisters gathered on the second floor of the convent in a recreation room where they were seated in wooden chairs facing a podium. Father Frank, a priest in his fifties, stood at the podium in traditional brown Franciscan robes and lectured in a jovial tone. The podium faced a closed-circuit video camera on the back wall. The lecture was a topic of conversation at meals for the following few days. Father Frank's lecture included an outline of the changes in prayer following Vatican II. During Vatican II, he said, the Vatican Council entirely reworked the rules of prayer for vowed members of the Church. The nuns had lived through all of this and knew well the changes he described.

In his lecture, Father Frank brought up the historical tradition of referring to God as "He." He noted that many modern prayer books, written in the past few decades, do not follow this pattern. In the following example, he rhetorically drilled the sisters about the subject of God's gender:

EXAMPLE 1: IS GOD A HE?
Participants
FF: Father Frank
SS: Sisters, in unison

01 FF: Is God a He?
02 SS: No.
03 FF: Is God a She?
04 SS: No.
05 FF: No! God's beyond that.
06   He and she are this big.
07   ((Makes one small circle in the air))

```
08        Here's a he, here's a she.
09        ((Makes two small circles in the air))
10        God is like this!
11        ((Motions with his arms in a huge circle in all
12        directions))
13        All right? God is He and She and They and It and
14        everything.
15        And all beauty and all goodness and beyond and
16        beyond and(.)
17        beyond.
```

Father Frank argued that by referring to God with a gendered pronoun (he), as was common before Vatican II, the divine was being contained or imagined as limited. Only by referring to God without these gendered pronouns, as has become more common since Vatican II, could one recognize the size and scope of the divine (lines 08–12). This new vision of God as "all beauty and all goodness and beyond" starkly contrasts than the vision of God portrayed by the Church in the centuries before Vatican II.

The prayer texts used in the convent before Vatican II indeed referred to the divine as a "He," as Father Frank pointed out. This male God was portrayed as an authority figure to be obeyed. In the pre–Vatican II days, the Franciscan Sisters of the Sacred Heart used a didactic prayer text by Adolphe Tanquerey, *The Spiritual Life*, published in English in 1930, which provided instructions on how to pray. The Franciscan Sisters of the Sacred Heart Convent, like many other convents in Europe and the United States, used this text through the first half of the twentieth century. In Tanquerey's 1930 prayer instructions, God is portrayed as a "Father" (e.g., 40–43), a "master" (e.g., 244–248), or a "benefactor" (e.g., 100, 244–245). The book emphasizes "humility" (200, 530–454) and "submission" (e.g., 243) and encourages readers to "elevat[e] [their] soul to God" (e.g., 243).

The nuns' daily prayers before Vatican II were consistent with Tanquerey's instructions on how to pray. For example, one of the daily prayers from the community prayer manual read, "Holy Father Saint Francis, keep me faithful to thy holy rule, obtain for me the spirit of sorrow in prayer, patience in trials, and purity in body and soul. . . . And let me copy from thee the spirit of obedience, humility and denial of self." These prayer directions characterized the divine as a male authority figure, and the text created an embodied map of the location of God in space in relation to humans. The divine was outside the human body. The nuns were encouraged to "bow before God," and the divine was described as "stoop[ing] down to us" (Tanquerey 1930, 243–252). As language and experience are interwoven, this repeated linguistic practice shaped the nuns' experiences in the world. This prayer process brought attention to their bodies as objects in space, below the divine, and as embodied persons in relationship with the divine. As the nuns repeated Tanquerey's words each day, they voiced and experienced Tanquerey's call to be humble before God, to bow to him, and to depend on him as a father, master, and benefactor. Sister Rita's narratives exemplify how these pre–Vatican II prayers were deeply incorporated into the nuns' embodied understanding of the divine.

Sister Rita, who joined the convent as a young woman in 1947, taught high school and worked as a hospital chaplain for years before retiring to the convent. In the narratives herein, she described her experience of an authoritative God before Vatican II, and she foreshadowed the changes that occurred after Vatican II. This first narrative will be contrasted with a second narrative that occurred later in my interview with her.

EXAMPLE 2: THE EYE OF GOD
Participants
SR: Sister Rita

```
01      So I went to the college then,
02      I was (.) put into (.) uh, classes for theology,
03      of which Church history was part.
04      I bega:n um: seeing that the Church was rather
05      rigid for me
06      It was pretty much just as our ho:me environment
07      was one of authority.
08      It was still in the Church.
09      They had not come to Vatican II yet.
10      Rather very legalistic,
11      and I would se:nse that,
12      as I did years later in a paper that I wrote,
13      that in my early days God was a judge
14      and He'd be up in some place
15      keeping track of what I was doing and when I was
16      good and when I was bad,
17      and it's h—int(h)er(h)esting because even when I
18      entered here in '47,
19      there was a picture in the dining room of an e:ye,
20      which is a symbol of the eye of God
21      and that you know
22      was that same image coming to me that indeed God
23      is watching us,
24      you know,
25      and I think the Church had not yet come out of
```

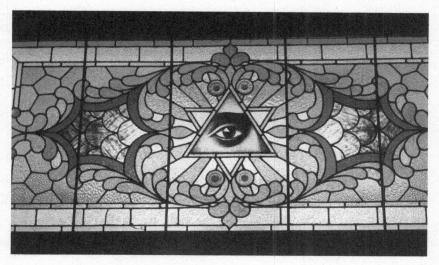

FIG. 5.3 The eye of God. (Photo by the author)

```
26      that shell
27      when I enter[ed], we lived a rather struct—
28      a very structured life.
```

In this first narrative, Sister Rita described God as a judge (line 13). She said that she pictured him "up" some place keeping track of her behavior (lines 14–16). In this description, Sister Rita positioned God as the surveyor and herself as the object of surveillance. She went on to describe a picture of the eye of God that was painted on the wall in the dining room, watching her (lines 19–23). This image still existed in the convent in a stained-glass window in the chapel when I was there (see fig. 5.3).

This image of God was one of a panopticon, an authoritative, omnipresent, all-seeing, and all-powerful judge in relation to which Sister Rita constructed her past self as an object of surveillance. She described a spatial distance between herself and the divine. This image of God is consistent with the characterization of God in Tanquerey's prayer books, where God is a "father" and "master" to whom individuals must bow down (1930). Sister Rita had read and repeated scripted prayers like Tanquerey's for the years between her entrance into the convent in 1947 until the transformation of prayer practices two decades later. Her experience of being surveilled by an authoritarian God above her corresponds to the practice of repeating scripted prayers, a practice structured by the Church that shaped her experience of the divine.

When I was in the convent, Vatican II was decades in the past; the sisters no longer read Tanquerey's books on prayer. Most of the sisters spent part of each day or week engaged in spiritual reading. They were free to choose books from the convent library, which had a number of shelves of books by contemporary Catholic authors. The most represented authors on the shelves included Joan Chittister, Thomas Merton, Henry Nouwen, and Joyce Rupp. In Rupp's book *Prayer*, there is a marked difference in how the divine is characterized and in the relationship she outlines for people to have with the divine. She never mentions God as a "father." Instead Rupp consistently refers to the divine as, simply, "God." She encourages "mutuality" (2007, 21–22), urging readers to "be with God" (e.g., 39) and to be in a "committed union with God" (11). Rupp writes that God is someone who "dwells within and among us" (14), who "breathes with us" (14). This description of God as "with" the reader, "dwelling within and among" her and "breathing" with her, creates a spatial proximity, even intermixing, between the individual and the divine (2007, 14). This close spatial proximity is in direct contrast to the spatial distance describe in Tanquerey's work, and in Sister Rita's image of God's eye looking down at her from above.

There is a distinct similarity between the description of God in Rupp's text and the nuns' descriptions of the divine after Vatican II, as is manifested in Sister Rita's second narrative:

EXAMPLE 3: DWELLING WITH GOD

Participants

SR: Sister Rita
AC: Anna Corwin (author)

```
01 AC   I would love to hear,
02      if you don't mind [a little more about] (.)
03      So, if God is no longer this authority figure,
04      how do you see God now?
05 SR   I'm glad you asked.
06      I see God for me (.) as my mother.
07      He is my belov'd (1.0),
08      and I see Go:d (.) as (.) no longer the judge (.),
09      no longer the eye (.),
10      but He lives within me (.)
11      and dwells within me (.)
12      and walks with me (.) when I go out.
13      There is a loving relationship. (.)
14      One of tenderness.
15      One of unity
16      and one that's accepting.
17      God for me is a God of love—
```

```
18        unconditional love.
19        He takes me as I am.
```

In this second narrative, Sister Rita described how she related to God decades after Vatican II. She described God as her "mother" (line 06), and, although this is clearly a female category, she continued to use male pronouns, saying in the next line that "He is my belov'd" (line 07). This relationship was one of "loving," "unity," and "tenderness" (lines 13–15). This description directly contrasted with the relationship described in the first narrative. Here, instead of constructing herself as the object of judgment and surveillance, Sister Rita was the implied daughter to God as a mother. She was the beloved partner to he who was her "belov'd."

Sister Rita's narratives show that she experienced a dramatic shift in her relationship with God after Vatican II. This shift is evidenced not only through the different descriptions of God outlined above but also through Sister Rita's linguistic performances of the two narratives. In these narratives Sister Rita not only represents two distinct relationships with the divine but also brings these contrastive relationships to life, performing them using distinct linguistic structures, cadence, genres, and spatial deixis, or markers. These are outlined in table 5.1.

Sister Rita's second narrative was performed with a number of rhetorical devices that made it more similar to poetic performance than ordinary conversational interaction. The first of these is parallelism that occurs in lines 10–12: "He lives within me / and dwells within me / and walks with me when I go out") and again in lines 13–16: "There is a loving relationship. / One of tenderness. / One of unity / and one that's accepting."). Parallelism occurs in poetry throughout the world and adds dramatic intensity to the speech or text (Jakobson 1987). As Max Atkinson has noted (1984), three-part lists, like the

Table 5.1
Genre of Sister Rita's narratives before and after Vatican II

	Before Vatican II	After Vatican II
<u>Genre</u>	Conversational	Biblical poetic form
Meter	Unmarked conversational prosody	Rhythmic, deliberate, slowed tempo
Lexicon	Standard English	Archaic English
Rhetorical devices	Simile ("Just as it was at home, it was still in the Church")	Grammatical and climactic parallelism
Heteroglossia	Quotes past self as author of paper	Revoices biblical passages

two in Sister Rita's narrative, are common in such public oratory as political speeches and are used as devices that strengthen the performance of a speaker's message.

Psalms, which are Biblical poems and hymns expressing thanksgiving and lament (Ralph 2003), use similar poetic devices. Parallelism in psalms can be seen to invoke the poetry of human breath and mimic the order of divine creation (Vos 2005). Sister Rita's use of parallel three-part lists made her second narrative distinct from the first with the effect that each line in the second narrative sounded like a verse from a poem in the genre of a biblical psalm. This genre was also evident in the lexicon of the second narrative: Sister Rita said that God "dwells within me" and "walks with me when I go out." These markers of the poetic biblical genre directly contrast the everyday conversational language of the first narrative. While the language of the second narrative is succinct and poetic, the first narrative is conversational.

Sister Rita also performed in this poetic genre through a distinct rhythm or cadence. The delivery of the second narrative was much slower and more rhythmic. She took a micropause at the end of each utterance to add poetic weight, and she systematically stressed certain words throughout the narrative. For example, she stressed the verbs in parallel lines 10–12—"He lives within me (.) / and dwells within me (.) / and walks with me (.)"—as well as the ultimate word in the utterance "when I go out," creating a poetic cadence not present in the first narrative. Through these performative features, Sister Rita not only described how God changed for her after Vatican II but embodied this change. She performed the relationship of unity and love that she experienced with poetic grace, channeling the affect, or emotion, of what she described. As she spoke, she exuded love, peace, and joy. Through the cadence, rhythm, and affect of her performance, Sister Rita embodied her loving and unified relationship with the divine. As her audience, I was moved by the narrative.

Finally, Sister Rita situated herself and the divine in space differently in each of the narratives; it was a spatial difference also present in the pre- and post-Vatican prayer books. In the first narrative, Sister Rita placed God as "up" somewhere, which placed her at a distance from the divine, looking up from below. After Vatican II, God was as close to Sister Rita as possible, mapped in space as next to her or within her body. In these two narratives, the divine had not just changed in character; God had also moved in the map of Sister Rita's lived space from a distant place above her to extreme proximity, existing within her. As this spatial relationship changed, Sister Rita herself moved from a place below the divine, looking up, to a place where she and God were together such that she was next to, or containing, him.

The notion of the divine "dwelling within" is not new to Catholicism. Saint Augustine stressed interiority as a means of experiencing God as early as the fourth century CE. But the nuns in the Franciscan Sisters of the Sacred Heart

Convent had little exposure to ideologies and prayer practices based upon this notion until the middle of the twentieth century. So while an emphasis on interiority was not new theologically, it was new to the nuns' everyday practices and their conceptions of the divine.

Sister Rita's embodied transformation mirrored that of Sister Theresa, who transitioned from seeing God as an arbiter of her suffering to a loving presence within her very body, existing even within the amoebas that plagued her. Sisters Theresa and Rita were not exceptional cases; the majority of the nuns in the Franciscan Sisters of the Sacred Heart Convent who lived through Vatican II described a similar shift, characterizing their experiences of the divine after Vatican II in more personal ways. As they understood and experienced God in these new ways, they experienced particular emotions, including love and spiritual unity.

The majority of the sisters at the convent described a similar amplification in their embodied experience of the divine following Vatican II. As the nuns prayed to a God who inhabited the space near them and in them, a God who emanated love and tenderness, they described themselves as being filled with the emotions of love, safety, and the knowledge that they were cared for by a benevolent companion. This new companionship, developed over decades, impacted the nuns' interpretation of their illnesses and chronic pain trajectories.

Suffering in the Convent

As Robert Orsi writes, Catholic ideologies and experiences of pain and suffering significantly transformed over the twentieth century. He explains that, before Vatican II, "pain purged and disciplined the ego, stripping it of pride and self-love; it disclosed the emptiness of the world" (2005, 21). Indeed, before Vatican II, the Franciscan Sisters of the Sacred Heart were encouraged to welcome pain and suffering as valuable resources to humble the ego. They were instructed to see their own pain and suffering as small reflections of the suffering Jesus endured for them. The nuns described pain and suffering as something they understood God required of them. Suffering was "offered up" to God. As they offered their suffering to the divine, they asked him to use their pain as he saw fit. The divine was seen to be the arbiter of their pain and suffering. As Sister Rita told me, suffering and pain were understood at that time as things God "wanted you to have." Through the process of offering up one's pain through prayer, the nuns created something virtuous out of their pain and suffering, but it was nevertheless seen as necessary punishment for the sins of humanity. Suffering and virtue were deeply connected for the nuns before Vatican II. Many Catholic convents have maintained a similar ideological connection between suffering and virtue since Vatican II. For example, Rebecca

Lester writes that postulants in a Mexican convent learned that suffering, albeit suffering with an "intention behind it" was the "path to sanctification" (2005, 194). This connection between pain and morality is not unique to Catholic cultural contexts (see, for example, Throop 2008). Since Vatican II, the Franciscan Sisters of the Sacred Heart have largely rejected the notion that suffering is virtuous or holy and have made an explicit effort to break this connection in their local ideologies and prayer practices.

In describing "old" ideologies of pain in the convent, Sister Rita said that the sisters used to think God "needed" human suffering in order to "be God." Now, she explained, they believe "just the opposite." She said, "God doesn't give us suffering. He's present in our suffering, but He certainly isn't doling it out." The concept of God's presence in one's suffering was key to the change that the sisters describe. While the pre–Vatican II God was the distant authoritarian who oversaw the distribution of pain and suffering to individuals in the world, for the Franciscan Sisters of the Sacred Heart, the post–Vatican II God became a close, supporting companion as they endured pain or suffering. As God moved "down" to "dwell within" them, the sisters came to experience him as a caregiver. Sister Rita described this relationship: "He goes with me throughout whatever it be. If it's pain, I know that He's there to support me. I think that that's a strong thing for our sisters, particularly in the infirmary, because, most of them have pain, of some type. And yet I marvel that they're not cranky, they're not complaining, um, they get wonderful care, which certainly helps them, but they're able as you say to somehow, God, Jesus, is very close to them. And He walks with them." Indeed, as Sister Rita described, the majority of the sisters in the infirmary, even those living with significant pain, used prayer and their relationship with the divine as a mode to garner comfort and support and to mitigate the pain they were experiencing. They also received robust social support from nursing staff and a significant team of sisters giving pastoral care who prayed with them and reminded them, as we saw with Sister Irma in chapter 3, that "Jesus loved them."

In pastoral care interactions in the infirmary, the sisters often called on the divine as a caregiver. Sister Irma regularly suggested that the sisters call on Jesus to comfort them, "walk with them," or "hold them." In one interaction, for example, she suggested that a sister who was suffering from tachycardia and anxiety should "relax" and "let Jesus hold you in His lap." Through this embodied directive, and others like it, she encouraged her fellow sisters to draw on the embodied presence of the divine to comfort them in times of need. The nuns' descriptions of their prayer experiences were varied. Some described prayer as a physical embrace with the divine; others described a more metaphorical "dwelling" together or copresence. Some of the nuns described detailed images. Sister Carline, for example, described an image of a teardrop held within a beautiful crystal goblet. She said that the teardrop represented her pain, suffering, and fear, and the goblet represented the beauty of God, which held her with love, representing the all-encompassing love and compassion of the divine. She described meditating on this image. Almost all of the sisters I interviewed described prayer practices in which they experienced a close proximity or complete envelopment of the divine within their own bodies.

As we have seen, after Vatican II the Franciscan Sisters of the Sacred Heart altered their cultural experience of pain and illness through their prayer practices. The "affective valences" (Throop 2008, 276) that the nuns associated with pain were no longer tied to virtue, suffering, and sin. Through the repeated practice of praying post–Vatican II prayer, pain for the sisters became affectively associated with God's supporting, calming presence. As they experienced pain and prayed with the divine, they experienced God as a caring, loving presence who "walked with them" and supported them. These new subjective states impacted the nuns' experiences of pain and illness by mitigating them or making them more bearable. In this way, institutional changes in prayer practices afforded new somatic patterns in the nuns' experiences of pain, illness, and old age. Pain ceased to carry the pre–Vatican II associations with a punishing God. Just as Sister Theresa was able to begin to love and forgive the amoebas infecting her body—seeing them as one with God, a loving, although perhaps difficult and painful presence—the majority of the sisters learned to accept their pain and call on God as a caring partner who helped them endure worldly suffering.

Summary: Transformation

Change in Catholic nuns' prayer lives has impacted religious sisters lives in many ways. Changes in prayer schedule has reordered their daily lives, and changes in the language and imagery of prayer have influenced their characterization of the divine. The nuns' understanding of God has been transformed from a male authority figure, located above the sisters looking down at them, to a more intimate companion, a being who resides next to them, supports them, and even exists within their bodies. This shift in the characterization of God has resulted in a new relationship with the divine. This changing notion of who God is and how the nuns relate to him has impacted more than their ideological relationship with God; it has also influenced their experiences of the world and their bodies and, ultimately, their ideologies and experiences of illness and chronic pain. David Morris argues that "pain is not just blindly felt or reflectively endured as a series of biochemical impulses. It changes with its place in human history" (1991, 45). The history of the Catholic Church as an institution has shaped the ways in which the nuns experience their bodies as they age.

The story of Vatican II is one in which institutional authorities and the individuals within the institution moved together in conversation to create profound change. Pope John XXIII responded to changing times and the work of various theologians to set in motion major institutional changes in the Church. Each convent was afforded its own interpretation and implementation of the changes. As prayer books were edited, and as local ideologies of the divine changed with them, Catholic nuns across the country had the opportunity to reshape their personal relationships with God. The change can be seen as coming both from the top down and from the bottom up.

Analysis of the nuns' narratives exemplifies the intimate connection between language and experience. As the nuns spoke new prayers, they experienced a new relationship with the divine. In Ochs's terms (2012), linguistic enactments were experienced as they were produced. The nuns' new prayer practices also integrated the body in new ways. Through a newly embodied relationship with the divine, they began to incorporate embodied prayer and ceased to emphasize the body as an object of prayer. For the nuns in the Franciscan Sisters of the Sacred Heart convent, changes in the words they spoke to God ultimately impacted their own interpretations and experiences of pain, suffering, and old age; how they moved through the world; how they responded to their aging bodies; and how they experienced the divine.

In chapter 6, which looks at ideologies of pain and healing and how they have transformed over time, we will see that some of the changes that came with historical changes in the Church and in the United States, both before and after Vatican II, are still being worked out. Some transformations, in other words, may still be underway.

6

Spiritual Healing,
Meaningful Decline, and
Sister Death

● ●

It was a cold sunny day, like many in the spring of 2011. Sister Carline sat reclined in a beige armchair in her room in the infirmary at the Franciscan Sisters of the Sacred Heart Convent. As usual, the shades were drawn, letting in only a dim light. Sister Carline and I had known each other for three years, since my first trip to the convent. A few weeks prior to this meeting, she had stopped her most recent round of chemotherapy and her gray hair was growing in downy soft, like a newborn's. She had me touch it, giggling at the pleasure of having hair again. Her face was gaunt, but her complexion had changed from the ashen hue of the past weeks. Her eyes were warm and kind, but her features maintained the etchings of significant pain and suffering.

Sister Carline was eighty-six, and this was her third serious bout with cancer. In the previous three decades, she had survived liver cancer and then ovarian cancer. Now she had uterine cancer. Her doctor had told her a few weeks earlier that the most recent round of chemotherapy had not been successful. After years of surgeries and chemotherapy, Sister Carline had decided not to try again. She understood that she would die in the next few months. Yet, in the quality of life questionnaire I distributed, Sister Carline responded that she only rarely felt depressed or nervous, and never sad. She, like most of the other nuns, reported that her life was overwhelmingly full with purpose, "worthwhile" and "complete." She reported feeling fully supported and had almost no fear of the future.

When I spoke to Sister Carline, she described her experience of physical pain and her thoughts on healing. Her discussion is representative of the many conversations I had with sisters in the infirmary wing of the convent. She spoke about accepting physical pain, describing it as an inevitability.

EXAMPLE 1: CONVERSATION WITH SISTER CARLINE, PART 1
SC: Sister Carline

```
01 SC:   You don't know what kind of pain you're gonna have,
02       how's it's gonna be.
03       You don't know when it's gonna be,
04       but you know it's on its way.
```

She described anticipating pain, but not fighting it or wishing it away. She told me that she did not pray for God to take away the pain. As we saw in chapter 5, the sisters I met saw God not as an arbiter of pain but as a companion in their pain. Sister Carline described an acceptance of pain as simply a part of life. When I asked how she was doing, she described her understanding of healing

```
05 SC:   I know that physical healing isn't gonna last forev—
06       it doesn't last forever for anybody,
07       but it's—
08       but me—
09       it's more imminent and
10       I know it's not gonna,
11       and I don't know how long it's gonna last.
12       . . .
13       We don't just have physical healing,
14       but the main kind of healing is spiritual healing;
15       you know that your whole body can accept whatever
16       is coming in your life.
```

Sister Carline accepted that even if she were to experience physical healing, that healing would not "last forever" (line 06). She described her understanding of the inevitability of death and the immediacy of her own mortality. Speaking both about healing and life, she said, "I don't know how long it's gonna last" (line 11); she understood that both would end in the near future. She followed this description of her impending mortality with a redirection away from an emphasis on "physical healing" (line 13), adding that "the main kind of healing is spiritual healing," which she defined as an acceptance by the "whole body" of "whatever is coming in life" (lines 14–16).

Sister Carline's narrative is complex and contradictory. She repeated the negative constructions "don't know" in a nearly poetic rendition of all that was unstable in her experiential world. She told me what she did not know, but then resolved this unknown in line 04 with what she did know, that the pain was "on its way." These fragmented renditions of what she did and did not know, that physical healing "isn't gonna last forever" (line 05), "doesn't last forever" (line 6), it is "not gonna [last]" (line 10) and "I don't know how long it's gonna last" (line 11) builds a tension in the narrative until, at last, in lines 14–16, Sister Carline produced a resolution: that spiritual healing was the "main kind of healing." In this moment, it seems, she was reminding herself, with sudden coherence, that her focus was on spiritual healing.

As I have established, the sisters experience significant positive health outcomes at the end of life. In what I have suggested is no coincidence, the nuns' ideologies of aging also run in contrast to the mainstream American model. This chapter looks at both of these elements as they relate to pain and healing as they were conceived in the convent. Later in the chapter we will look closely at another intricate passage from Sister Carline in which contrasting ideas about pain and healing emerge. This is a complicated story to analyze. Unlike the transition from one prayer practice to another that we traced in chapter 5, the sisters' notions of pain, illness, and healing are products of multiple intertwining cultural histories. In this chapter, I attempt to trace the complex and intertwined cultural meanings of pain, illness, and healing as they emerge in the nuns' lives. I do not provide complete histories here, as such a task would require many books, but I do attempt to untangle the multiple cultural histories as they emerge in the convent to shape the sisters' experiences of aging and the body.

I will suggest that the complex histories of pain in the Catholic Church, as they are filtered through the institution of this particular convent along with contemporary medical models of pain, convene to render a complex and often contradictory model of pain and healing that the nuns themselves are continuing to make sense of even as they experience them. As complex and perhaps unresolved as this is, it is an important element of the nuns' experiences of aging. If we wish to understand the nuns' aging trajectories, we must also examine the elements of their lives that are less coherent or tidy since, too, have influenced how they have aged.

We all live with tensions and contradictions in our lives. Yet when we tell our everyday narratives, we often tidy up these tensions and contradictions to present singular coherent stories. As Elinor Ochs and Lisa Capps write, narratives "imbue life events with a temporal or logical order, to demystify them and establish coherence across past, present, and as yet unrealized experience" (2001, 2). The world does not come to us packaged into coherent stories. Life is messy, filled with seemingly infinite detail. It is through the process of narrating our lives to ourselves and others that we bring coherence to an otherwise disorganized world.

Occasionally we encounter narratives that are themselves incoherent and messy. When this happens, it can indicate that something very interesting is at work. This chapter will look at how Sister Carline's complex narrative is tied to intertwining cultural histories to reveal how they impact the sisters' aging trajectories. We will see that much as the sisters' model of aging contrasts the contemporary American paradigm, the story of pain here contradicts contemporary secular models of pain and illness.

The notion of spiritual healing that Sister Carline introduces is interesting in a few ways. First, it echoes historical Catholic ideologies about pain in which physical suffering offers a pathway to spiritual purity. Second, it speaks to a historical orientation to pain as normative. As we will see a little later in the chapter, medical interventions now provide significant options for the alleviation of pain. Sister Carline's orientation to pain as normative rather than as a moral or medical problem resonates with how the Catholic Church has seen pain for centuries. The notion of spiritual healing also echoes a theme in Christianity in which pain offered the possibility for intersubjective union with the divine. After a brief look into the history of pain in the Church, we will return to Sister Carline's experience to examine how the complex histories of pain and illness in the Church and in Western medicine have shaped the nuns' experiences of their bodies and their conceptions of pain and decline.

The Body in the Church

In the Catholic Church, the body has been understood to be a site of vulnerability, representing a pathway to sin. Bodily desires, such as for food or sex, have often been framed in Catholic settings as dangerous temptations that can contaminate the soul (Lester 2005, 35). Through discipline, however, the body has been understood to be a vessel through which one can achieve spiritual purity. In contrast to some protestant Christian models, such as contemporary evangelical Christianity, which presents the notion that internal sincerity will lead to closeness to God and purity of soul (Ikeuchi 2017, Shoaps 2002), Catholicism has historically presented a model in which ritual behavior is understood to transform the individual through ritual forms. These ritual forms include physical discipline—for example, kneeling on wooden planks in prayer or spending entire nights without sleep as one prays in the presence of the Holy Sacrament. In Catholicism, the physical form of prayer—through scripted texts and actions—is understood to align the self with the divine. Like Buddhist monasticism (Cook 2001) and Japanese practices of both Buddhism and Shinto (Ikeuchi 2017), Catholicism emphasizes the role of ritual form in shaping the individual. Form has been understood in the Church, and particularly in monastic contexts, as the pathway to purification. As we saw in chapter 5, bodily forms—such as how one dresses, prays, eats, or walks—were strictly monitored in the Franciscan Sisters of the Sacred Heart Convent before Vatican II. The nuns understood that if they engaged in specific behaviors, such as praying proscribed prayers at proscribed times, abiding by monastic rules, and dressing in the habit, they would be spiritually transformed.

In their first years at the convent, the postulants and novices repeated prayers to remind them that their bodies were vessels of spiritual purity and oneness with God. As a symbolic pathway toward spiritual purity, however, the body could also pose problems. Since the body and its actions could lead a person either to spiritual purity or to its opposite, sin, the body and its desires were treated with care. Pain was a particularly rich site for this type of meaning making.

Pain: Communion with God, or a Medical Problem?

In medical settings in North America and around the world, pain is understood to be an embodied indication that something has gone wrong. In other words, pain is a problem. It is undesirable. In a biomedical context, pain is understood to be a negative experience and there is an expectation that one should work to resolve or alleviate it. Pain can be an index of an underlying problem, as in a symptom of a disorder that can be diagnosed and treated. Unexplainable pain, without an identified underlying cause, can itself be a problem—hence the use of painkillers and therapies. Historically and cross-culturally, however, pain has not been universally understood to be bad. Just as Sister Theresa demonstrated in chapter 5, when she addressed the amoebas in her body as God within herself, pain and illness can be interpreted in multiple ways. Chris Shilling and Philip Mellor write that pain has been associated with various meanings historically, "ranging from ideas of legal punishment (e.g. 'on pain of death'), to having one's belief tested by God." They describe the novelty of the scientific medical paradigm, which has "restricted pain to this-worldly issues of sensation, location, measurement, and control" (2010, 523).

Pain does not always or only represent evidence of a problem. Anthropological literature on initiation rituals, which take place in communities around the world and involve the infliction of heightened pain through a controlled ritual process, have found that individuals engaging in initiation rituals understand the pain in ways that contrast the biomedical model. For example, initiation rituals are experienced by individuals not as problematic but as symbolically meaningful. Alan Morinis writes that in the context of an initiation ritual, the "excruciating ordeal creates a peak experience which in turn results in an intensification of personal self-awareness. By heightening self-awareness, pain exaggerates the opposition between the self and society in the minds of initiands." He suggests that the pain of initiation is sometimes understood to move the initiand toward "adult consciousness" and is understood as indexical of the weight of psychological and social transformation (1985, 171). Others have suggested that pain can serve to sever ties with the nuclear family and to create a sense of bonding and identification with other adult men (Whiting, Kluckhohn, and Anthony 1958). In experimental settings, shared experiences of pain, such as the experience of having one's hands submerged in ice water, enduring leg squats, or eating hot chili peppers, have been found to increase social bonding and cooperation (Bastian, Jetten, and Ferris 2014, 2079). These results echo theories of social bonding and cohesion presented over a century earlier by Émile Durkheim (1912).

Although pain is universal—no human lives without experiencing pain at some point, pain itself can change shape and meaning across contexts. Jason Throop writes that pain "may be transformed through the particular meanings, values, ideas and expectations that we bring to bear in dealing with the existential possibilities and limitations that it evokes." As such, "pain is variegated in its forms of manifestation and significance" (2010, 2). The diversity of approaches to pain and the possibility that pain can be understood differently across cultural settings reveals a few things. First, it reveals that the notion of pain as a problem is a cultural orientation. This orientation is neither a fixed "truth" nor an objective "fact." Even within mainstream American settings, we can see evidence of this diversity. For example, pain in childbirth or during strenuous exercise can be seen as meaningful or positive. Second, this diversity demonstrates that the meaning pain holds is learned through social processes that unfold over time (Good et al. 1994; McGrath 1990; Morris 1991; Pincikowski 2013). Finally, it reveals that the ways in which we understand pain can shape how we experience it. Pain is not one thing; it can be many different things and can lead to many possible experiences and interpretations.

Pain in the Catholic Church

Historically, the Catholic Church and the Bible have portrayed pain as a saving force, one that could render individuals spiritually pure. In the book of Romans, suffering is presented as morally valuable: "We rejoice in our sufferings, knowing that suffering produces endurance, and endurance produces character, and character produces hope" (5:3–4). In the church, pain was understood not as a trial from God but simply a fact of human life. For early Christians, suffering "confirmed their belief that they were part of Christ's Church" (Hauerwas 2004, 84). Following the theme of Christ's resurrection, pain emerged as a vehicle for salvation and unity with Christ, who also endured suffering and, through Christ, God's connection with humans. In the early Church, pain and suffering were understood as a given, an accepted part of life.

The role of religion was not to explain or remediate pain and suffering but, given the inevitability of suffering to the human condition, to build communities of support within the Church (Swinton 2007, 35).

On the broader topic of "evil," a theological name for causes of suffering, Stanley Hauerwas writes, "Historically speaking, Christians have not had a 'solution' to the problem of evil. Rather, they have had a community of care that has made it possible for them to absorb the destructive terror of evil that constantly threatens to destroy all human relations" (2004, 49). Although suffering has been integral to Christian life since its inception (Hauerwas 2004, 84), the interpretations of suffering and pain have changed over time. One large-scale change in the interpretation of pain arose with technological advances in medicine when it became increasingly possible to alleviate pain. Rather than a vehicle for salvation, pain has since been reconceived as an indication of a problem, an experience that could—and eventually should—be avoided. As Shilling and Mellor write, "Western culture has moved from the belief that the world could be saved through pain, as represented by certain early Christian and by late medieval Christian orientations, to one where it is believed that the world can be saved from pain" (2010, 533). This change is rooted in both Enlightenment thinking and advances in medical technologies that have afforded the possibility of pain avoidance and alleviation. Historically, the "self-in-pain" was "normative [to a] Christian identity," while in later centuries, "the pain-free self," a relatively new possibility, has become, in Shilling and Mellor's words, "a model of contemporary productivity" (2010, 522). As Catholic theologian John Swinton writes, "increasing successes in medicine bring with them increased expectations that suffering should no longer be a part of our experience" (2007, 38).

It is important to remember that this orientation toward pain is very new. Historically, the Catholic Church conceptualized pain as normative, as bearable, and as a path toward salvation: "As early as the second century, . . . Christianity developed an emerging view of the human self as a body in pain; facilitating religious explorations of how believers could not just bear pain, or be cured of pain, but could be saved through pain" (Shilling and Mellor 2010, 527; see also Perkins 2002). Early Christian texts such as the Apocryphal Acts of the Apostles, which depict the lives of John, Peter, Paul, Andrew, and Thomas, portray pain as "the means to Christian salvation" (Shilling and Mellor 2010, 528). Early Christianity portrayed pain as a normative accepted part of life and as a means for salvation after death.

Stephen Greenblatt connects the Christian orientation to pain to pre-Christian Roman cultural orientations to pain. Romans, known for celebrating bravery and endurance in battle and in brutal spectacles such as those in the gladiators' arena, saw the voluntary acceptance of pain as a marker of courage and endurance. Greenblatt suggests that early Christianity "offered a moralized and purified version of the Roman pain principle" (2011, 104). He goes on to posit that, in this context, pleasure—which had been embraced, particularly by Romans influenced by Greek Stoicism—also took on new meaning:

> Early Christians, brooding on the sufferings of the Savior, the sinfulness of mankind, and the anger of a just Father, found the attempt to cultivate pleasure manifestly absurd and dangerous. At best a trivial distraction, pleasure was at worst a demonic trap.... The only life truly worth imitating—the life of Jesus—bore ample witness to the inescapable presence in mortal existence of sadness and pain, but not of pleasure.... As every pious reader of Luke's Gospel knew, Jesus wept, but there were no versus that described him laughing or smiling, let alone pursuing pleasure." (Greenblatt 2011, 105)

This orientation toward pleasure as problematic and pain as purifying is exemplified in an anecdote preserved by Pope Gregory I, or Gregory the Great, in his *Dialogues* written about Saint Benedict (ca. 594). Saint Benedict, the author of *The Rule of Saint Benedict*, was influential in shaping Christian monasticism, and the rule was used as a model for many other monastic communities. The following story from Pope Gregory's *Dialogues* describes Saint Benedict's desire to avoid pleasure, seen as temptation sent by the devil, and his intentional use of bodily pain as means of purification. Saint Benedict was so disturbed by a memory, which recalled temptation into sexual pleasure, that he quashed the memory of pleasure by seeking out the purifying force of bodily pain:

> One day when the Saint was alone, the Tempter came in the form of a little blackbird, which began to flutter in front of his face. It kept so close that he could easily have caught it with his hand. Instead, he made the sign of the cross and the bird flew away. The moment it left, he was seized with an unusually violent temptation. The evil spirit called to his mind a woman he had once seen, and before he realized it, his emotions were carrying him away.... He then noticed a thick patch of nettles and briars next to him. Throwing his garment aside he flung himself into the sharp thorns and stinging nettles. There he rolled and tossed until his whole body was in pain and covered with blood. Yet, once he had conquered pleasure through suffering, his torn and bleeding skin served to drain the poison of temptation from his body. Before long, the pain was burning his whole body and had put out the fires of evil in his heart. It was by exchanging these two fires that he gained victory over sin. (Saint Gregory the Great 2011, 59–60)

We see here that worldly pleasure, first in the form of a blackbird and then in the form of a memory of a woman to whom he was sexually attracted, was problematic for Saint Benedict. In this account, the threat of this pleasure was so morally problematic that he took great measures to eliminate it. Saint Gregory describes in detail the purifying force of physical pain as Saint Benedict is reported to have inflicted pain on himself to "gain victory over sin." Pain was both meaningful and purifying in this context.

Julian of Norwich, the first female mystic whose writings have been preserved, inherited this tradition. She lived in the fourteenth century as an anchorite, residing in a cell attached to a church. As was customary practice for anchorites, after she moved into the cell the door was sealed closed with mortar. She lived the rest of her days bricked in, with only a window into the church to receive Communion and a small window to the garden where a servant would deliver her meals and remove her waste. Christ's suffering held particular emotional and moral significance for Julian; she wanted nothing more than to experience pain and suffering, as he had experienced it. She prayed that she might experience a fragment of his suffering. According to her writing, her prayers were answered. She became extremely ill and, following a painful near-death experience, had visions of Christ. She recorded the mystical fulfillment of her prayers as she witnessed Christ's passion, seeing his "red blood trickling down from under the crown of thorns" (Julian of Norwich 1998, 45). She prayed that she might have a vision of Christ on the crucifix and see "his face covered . . . in dry blood . . . blood coming from the weals from the scourging." In a vision, she saw "his face dry and bloodless with the pallor of death . . . ashen and exhausted (as it) went blue, then darker blue, as the flesh mortified more completely" (1998, 15).

To a contemporary audience, Julian's orientation toward pain may be unintuitive. She intentionally *chose* to become ill and to suffer. She wanted to experience physical pain and to witness Christ's pain. Her spiritual journey only makes sense if we understand medieval European orientations toward pain and illness, in which pain was understood to "fuse the body and soul into one" (Lichtmann 1991, 9). As Maria Lichtmann writes, "A suffering that is willed, desired, and actively chosen as was Julian's, as part of a larger context of meaning and purpose, is transformed into something more. . . . Like Teresa of Avila, Julian goes from living on the surface—an aimless, slothful, frivolous life—to living at the depth and center of her soul" (1991, 9). Julian writes that pain is a penance, one that "we ought to bear and suffer the penance which God himself gives us" (1998, 330). Pain, here, is a moral obligation to God, one that allows for a transformation of the soul; it is also a means to connect and experience compassion with other beings. As Lichtmann notes, "Julian's bodily experience, her sickness and her body wounded with compassion, may well be the link between her suffering, Christ's suffering, and a compassionate feeling of oneness with all other beings" (1991, 14). As a mode of compassion and connection with others, pain had been merged over the centuries with expressions of love in the Catholic tradition. For medieval practitioners like Julian, pain held the power to unite individuals with the divine. Embodied suffering had the power to transform the soul and to purify the individual as the individual united with God.

The divine's embodied suffering can also be seen as a move toward radical empathy, a unique form of intersubjectivity. Julian of Norwich described her visions as rendering God—who, at first, was separate from her—"familiar" and "intimate" to her. When Christ manifested in her visions as a human who suffered pain in a human body, just as she suffered pain in a human body, he became intersubjectively available to her in new ways. Connecting with Jesus seems to have allowed Julian, as well as the Franciscan Sisters of the Sacred Heart, to imagine the divine as deeply human (like they are), having a body (like they have), and suffering (as they have suffered). In the convent, the radical empathy of God functioned to bring the divine into a proximate space—a here and now—that allowed the sisters to feel a personal, intersubjective connection with the divine. In other words, Jesus's pain, which was like their pain, and his body, which was like their bodies, rendered him relatable and intersubjectively available. Through this intimate connection with the divine, a transformation could take place.

Many of the nuns' prayer practices revolved around a similar cultivation of intersubjectivity with the divine. Sister Betsy, for example, whom we met in chapter 2, would gaze for hours each day at a drawing of Christ with the crown of thorns, droplets of red blood trickling down his forehead. She told me that as she looked at his face she would repeat the words "Jesus, Jesus, Jesus" while concentrating on a sense of love and devotion. Sister Mary Augusta told me that that each time she passed a large statue of the crucifixion, she would imagine Jesus embracing her with his arms around her and hers around him.

When the sisters whom I met in the infirmary first joined the Franciscan Sisters of the Sacred Heart Convent, the Church had moved away from medieval models in which pain was intentionally invited or inflicted as a means for purification of the soul. Yet they were still taught that pain was a sacrament and that offering up one's pain through prayer had the potential to purify the soul and achieve good in the world. This was a delicate balance: although pain was understood as a form of unity with God and as integral to Christian lives, it was nevertheless not to be invited (Hauerwas 2004, 84). Sister Betsy, who endured chronic pain, was taught to offer her pain up to God to atone for her sins, and she experienced the pain as a way to connect with the divine. Despite this model of pain as a form of devotion and connection, Sister Betsy was warned never to want pain or to invite it as Julian of Norwich did. This was a delicate paradox made more complex by biomedical understandings of pain.

Pain and Medicine

Until the mid-nineteenth century, nursing was not a healing-oriented project. Pain and suffering were understood not as indicators of medically remediable problems but as signs of moral transgression. Illness was often understood to be an indicator of sin. Historians of nursing Carol Helmstadter and Judith Godden write that in eighteenth- and nineteenth-century Europe, "disease was identified with sin, or a visitation from God to improve the moral character of the sick person," They write that nurses were known to whip and admonish patients before releasing them in an effort to prevent them from sinning again (2016, 4). It was not until the secularization of hospitals, which involved hospitals' integration with medical doctors, that this orientation to pain was replaced. The advent of medical technology in the mid-1800s created an environment in which pain could be treated and suffering became antithetical to medical healing (Soine 2009).

In her work on early hospice care, Joy Buck writes that at the turn of the nineteenth century, when physical cures were not achievable, nurses focused on "soul cures" that relied on the patient's acceptance of Christian ideals. She writes, "Although spiritual healing was paramount, it was generally accepted that this could not be accomplished until the person's physical and mental suffering had been alleviated. . . . The hospices emphasized the importance of 'being with' patients through their final hours and attended to their individual needs" (2006, 115, 118). The response to suffering that Buck describes here, where a caregiver's goal was to "be with" those who were suffering, to provide comfort but not a solution, contrasts with the contemporary biomedical approach to pain and suffering. As Shilling and Mellor write, in medical contexts pain and suffering are problems to be solved: "The contemporary Western approach towards pain is characterized by instrumentalization—the reduction of pain to a manageable, technical phenomenon—and key to this is the process of medicalization." They see this process as incorporating two steps. Citing David Morris (1999, 22–23), Rebecca Sachs Norris (2009, 23) and Scott Pincikowski (2002, 3), they write that first, "medically identified pain became a phenomenon to be avoided if not eradicated through pain relief." Following this, Shilling and Mellor add, "One by-product of this medical colonization was that it became difficult to approach the experiential dimensions of pain outside the parameters of aversion and avoidance" (2010, 523). In this new paradigm, nurses and physicians were tasked with the goal of eliminating pain and illness. The failure to eliminate pain became an indication of the limits or failure of the medical system itself. In this new symbolic arrangement, where the success of the medical system depended on the successful eradication of pain and suffering, pain was no longer seen to be a normal part of life and certainly was not a sacrament or meaningful pathway to God. Instead, pain emerged in the contemporary era as an indication of institutional or personal failure.

Immersed in both Catholic theological tradition and the biomedical model of healing, the Franciscan Sisters of the Heart navigate a complex landscape. On the one hand, the Catholic Church has a historical relationship with pain that rendered pain meaningful, transformative, and a way to commune with the divine. On the other hand, the nuns live in the twenty-first century in the United States, where the medical paradigm interprets suffering to be at best a useful indicator of a problem to be fixed and, at worst, an indication of physical or institutional failure if it cannot be fixed, such as in the case of terminal illness.[1]

In this context the intrinsic contradictions in Sister Carline's narrative begin to reveal a historical logic. In the convent, managing healing and illness carry complex cultural histories that bring together deep and changing Catholic traditions with North American biomedical traditions. Pain has complex theological meanings that change over time. When I met the nuns, the nuns understood pain, like aging, to be a normal part of life, and God's role was to "walk with" or support the sisters in their pain. The nuns praised God if they were healed, but they did not ask to be healed. Similarly, they were expected to accept what came and not to expect or take advantage of God's power to heal.

As Americans, accessing medical care is a normal part of life. The nuns have regular doctors' appointments and medicine is a normative, accepted technology available to them. For the nuns, medicine exemplifies the potential of God's saving power.[2] For example, when I met Sister Carline in 2008, chemotherapy had successfully treated her first two bouts of cancer. When she relayed this at the time, she expressed gratitude to God. She understood God's will to be integral to the chemotherapy's success. But celebrating God's capacity to heal or "save" did not mean that the nuns accepted the biomedical model's orientation toward death or chronicity as moral failures. As we have seen, nuns like Sister Carline accepted decline and death as also part of God's will. In chapter 7 we will explore how this acceptance of health and decline connects to the nuns' vow of obedience.

Medical care represents both the healing power God made available to (and through) humans and an "intervention" that at times is understood to contrast with the sisters' vows of obedience and poverty. To cling to medical intervention to such an extent that one does not accept God's will is understood as contradicting the vow of obedience. For instance, when the chemotherapy did not work for Sister Carline's cancer in 2011, her vow of obedience, which required accepting God's will, dictated that she should accept that it was her time rather than ask her doctor to try again. Similarly, for a nun to ask the convent to spend too much money on medical interventions would contradict her vow of poverty. The cost of medical care could therefore present a moral dilemma. More than once, I heard some of the institutional authorities in the convent suggest that the older sisters were unaware of how much it cost the convent to provide the medical care they were given. I heard sisters suggest that they should be more conservative with their trips to the doctor. Another sister said that her older peers were getting too comfortable with "Cadillac medical care," adding, "We're Franciscan, after all," meaning that as Franciscans who have made a commitment to a life of poverty, it was not appropriate to expect expensive medical care if it placed undue financial burden on the community. This was an increasingly pertinent conversation, since the convent was financially dependent on the working nuns' wages, and the median age of the nuns continued to rise because fewer and fewer novices had been joining the convent in recent decades.

For the sisters, a desire to avoid pain and illness was both morally "right" and could be antithetical to their ethical orientation to the world. Paying for expensive health care was seen as indulgent, and the act of praying for healing could threaten one's reliance on divine authority. Nevertheless, to not accept a medical "saving" of the body, or to not go to the doctor, would similarly flout God's saving power. The nuns thus navigated a paradox: saving the body and maintaining health while simultaneously accepting the body's decline. Most sisters managed to walk this delicate path with grace. Instead of seeking "saving" through bodily health, like Sister Carline, the nuns strived for spiritual healing, which entailed accepting God's will. It was this actively cultivated sense of acceptance that allowed them to embrace aging.

Returning to Sister Carline

At the beginning of the chapter, we saw how Sister Carline struggled to express her attitude toward death and suffering. On one hand, she said she strived to accept death and saw terminal cancer as something that God had "allowed" to happen or perhaps had created. She saw death as part of a trajectory that God was in charge of, and she strived to "befriend" death as she understood Saint Francis to have done. At the same time, Sister Carline did not want to assume she would die nor did she want death (or, at least, she did not want to be seen as longing to die). To assume that her death was imminent would defy God's saving power and the possibility of miracles. To want death would disrespect the life God had given her thus far.

In her narrative, we see Sister Carline trying to navigate this paradox: accepting illness and death while also not *wanting* it. The text below is a long passage, but I encourage the reader to take the time to read it, as it gives us insight into Sister Carline's complex internal experience.

EXAMPLE 2: CONVERSATION WITH SISTER CARLINE, PART 2

SC: Sister Carline
AC: Anna Corwin (author)

01 SC: I really feel like that peace is deeper,
02   you know, than in the beginning,
03   because I kept praying
04   and I kept praying it, and,
05   and sometimes I'd be just you know kind of you know,
06   I—not—**not resisting** but kind of **struggling** with it.
07   And so as time as been going on, you know,
08   **I do feel more peace** with where I am,
09   you know,
10   knowing that I feel like God's peace has been
11   given to me,
12   and, and I'm praying that it even goes deeper,
13   you know, that it just keeps going so,
14   **I don't want to be struggling, I want to—**
15   **I want** to welcome,
16   **want** to welcome death,
17   and it's really, you know, like all the scripture
18   and everything say,
19   it's really **not a death,**
20   **it's really going from life to life.**
21   This life to the next life,
22   so the death is like, *psssst*, you know,
23   just a second
24   but you continue to live,
25   but you live in a different form a different
26   atmosphere, and, so,
27   **I try to,**
28   that's what **I try to do**: befriend,
29   befriend like Saint Francis always called 'em,
30   Sister Death, Sister Death, Brother Sun,
31   Sister Moon, and all that.
32   But he always—sister—and I thought, you know,
33   that's a good way to think,
34   **to welcome that rather than to fight it.**
35   You know, because when you fight something it's
36   more painful and the **struggle** is worse.
37   So **if I can** just *surrender*,
38   I think that's the word I've used most,

39 you know, to surrender, um,

40 so that **I would** be able to accept whatever comes,

41 because, you know, you don't know what kind of

42 pain you're gonna have,

43 how's it's gonna be,

44 you don't know when it's gonna be,

45 but you know it's on its way.

46 And, um,

47 so I just, uh, keep that in mind and kind of keep

48 myself living,

49 you know, live as long as we live, and **I want** to

50 live fully.

51 **I don't want** to [be] haphazard or, you know, just

52 groaning around, you know,

53 **I want** it to be a full life as long as I'm living

54 and happy life, you know . . .

55 I do think that, well, you read many times that

56 laughter is healing, and even though

57 I know that physical **healing isn't gonna last**

58 **forev—,**

59 **it doesn't last forever** for anybody,

60 but it's,

61 but me,

62 it's more imminent and

63 **I know it's not** gonna, and **I don't know** how long

64 it's gonna last.

65 **But I wanna** keep that sense of humor, and going,

66 and that,

67 that <u>**we don't just have physical healing.**</u>

68 <u>**But the main kind of healing is spiritual healing**</u>,

69 you know, that your whole body can accept whatever

70 is coming in your life, and

71 um, you know

72 if somebody says **do you want** to die,

73 no **I don't want** to die,

74 I mean, you know, **it's not that I'm craving to die**

75 **although sometimes,**

76 **sometimes when you're feeling kind of sick**

77 **or, you know, you don't feel good**

78 **you thought, Oh, maybe that's not gonna be so bad,**

79 **you know?**

80 AC: Yeah.

```
81  SC:   But it's not that I'm, uh, you know, sitting here
82        waiting to die, but
83        I'm gonna take when it comes,
84        you know,
85        I want to be ready to hand it over,
86        to surrender when that time comes.
```

Sister Carline's narrative contains multiple contradictions: she was not "resisting" pain, but she was "struggling" with it (line 06); she was struggling, but she did not "want to be struggling" (line 14); she was not "craving" to die, but she admitted that it would not be so bad (lines 72–79); she wanted to welcome death, but pointed out that death was not actually death; death was going from "life to life" (line 20). In the end, she resolved these recursive paradoxes with the statement that she wanted "to be ready to hand it over, to surrender when that time comes" (lines 85–86). This notion of surrender permeated her narrative, offering a relief to the tension created by the recursive paradoxes. At each turn, she suggested that surrender was the only solution. In lines 37–40, she used the subjunctive tense: "So if I can just *surrender* / I think that's the word I've used most, / you know, to surrender, um, / so that I would be able to accept whatever comes." Here she suggested that surrender would allow her to accept all permutations of her possible futures. Surrender (meaning surrendering to God's will) would allow her to let go and experience peace. Sister Carline's conclusion echoes Sister Joan Chittister's description of aging in her book *The Gift of Years: Growing Older Gracefully*: "It's time now for surrender to acceptance. Perhaps for the first time in our adult lives we will go into a period of total dependence. . . . This is the time for melting into God. . . . The veil between us and eternity will begin to tear and we will begin the slow walk through it, ready, open, thrown upon the heart of God" (2010, 222).

In her discussion of the vow of obedience, Rebecca Lester writes, "The sisters believe that from the moment they surrender themselves to blind obedience—totally renouncing their liberty, never more belonging to the world—they will be free" (2005, 76). This aspiration to surrender rather than to strictly avoid pain sets the nuns apart from mainstream American aging trajectories. Instead of desiring relief exclusively through bodily health and resolution from pain, the sisters I met strived for spiritual healing or saving of the soul, which entailed accepting God's will. This cultivated sense of being spiritually "saved" required accepting death and decline.

In the United States, the popular discourse on aging, health, and medicine suggests that a successful medical trajectory is to resist death, to fight diseases (Martin 1994). As we saw in chapter 2, the contemporary discourses on aging present the notion that "successful" aging involves independence, productivity, agelessness, and avoidance of death and decline. In contrast, in the convent pain could be interpreted as a sign of a medical problem, but chronic or untreatable pain, along with notions of aging, decline, and death, were not interpreted as medical or moral failings. To be ill, to age, and to experience pain was not seen as a medical or moral failure. And pain had meaning. As Rebecca Sachs Norris writes, "in a context where pain and suffering are not understood to have value, that attitude can create more suffering, even in conditions meant to alleviate suffering, such as in biomedical situations" (2009, 22). She suggests here that if pain and suffering have no value, as in many medical settings, this can create more suffering for individuals who are experiencing pain. Norris writes, however, that "in contrast, where pain and suffering are understood to be valuable, such as within a religious context, those experiences can be used for spiritual transformation; the liminal state that pain can induce contributes to this process" (2009, 22). The Sisters of the Sacred Heart inhabited an ideological landscape in which pain was no longer seen as a tool to be harnessed to create spiritual transformation. They no longer wore woolen habits in the humid summer heat; they no longer knelt during Mass, as it hurt their knees. Pain was no longer an instrument used to create meaning. Yet the nuns maintained a sense that pain was meaningful. Suffering afforded an opportunity for God to accompany them in their pain, a possibility for closeness with the divine and support and intimacy from the community as they endured pain, but it was no longer a tool directly employed to create closeness with God. Age-related decline and chronic conditions were not moral or medical failings. They were opportunities to be in communion with God.

Summary: Pain as Spiritual Healing

The intertwining ideologies of pain we have witnessed in Sister Carline's narrative are a result of a transformation that Sister Carline and her peers are still undergoing. They are engaged in a process that is still unfolding in time. These changes may continue to unfold in the coming decades. Unlike their Christian predecessors, the nuns I met did not value pain to an extent that they sought it out. No one was rolling in briars and nettles to quell temptation, as Saint Benedict was reported to have done. Yet the sisters did not see pain and illness as "failures" or "valueless," as the contemporary biomedical model often does. The nuns readily sought out medical interventions when medicine could be directly useful, as Sister Carline did with chemotherapy, but they also understood that the biomedical relationship with pain had its limits. Here the sisters maintained the theological notion that pain and illness are inevitable parts of the human condition that can bring a person into meaningful communion with the divine. This combination of cultural orientations created a landscape in which the nuns were able to accept pain. It was an inevitable element of human existence that, when accepted, could bring one closer to God. In Sister Carline's words, it was an opportunity for "spiritual healing." This orientation to pain afforded an attitude in which decline and death could be accepted and also meaningful.

7

Kenosis

•••••••••••••••••••••

Emptying the Self

Although Sister Carline had to endure the embodied and psychic suffering of cancer, cancer treatment, and the inevitability of her own mortality, she handled all of it with remarkable equanimity and grace. When David Snowdon published his popular book on his findings from this well-known epidemiological study of nuns (2001), he titled it *Aging with Grace*. Each time I walked into Sister Carline's room, Snowdon's phrase echoed in my head. The concept of grace evokes two things: first, grace references gracefulness, as in to age or to move gracefully. Indeed, many of the nuns were moving through time, aging, in a graceful manner and with serenity, peace, and kindness. The notion of grace also invokes the concept of the Holy Spirit or Holy Ghost, one part of the Holy Trinity that makes up the divine for Christians. The Trinity, which is understood to be both tripartite and a singular God, is made up of the Father, God in heaven; the Son, Jesus Christ, the human embodiment of God; and the Holy Ghost, the essence of the divine. Worldly operations of grace are attributed to the Holy Ghost. For the Franciscan Sisters of the Sacred Heart, the Holy Spirit was understood to be the ineffable sense of holiness or spirituality embodied in all things. The concept of aging with grace conjures not only the nuns' actions as they moved forward in time but also suggests that the nuns were aging with God—specifically, the Holy Spirit, the essence of the divine, which they had witnessed, absorbed, and enacted throughout their lives and now experienced at the very end.

Sister Carline and many of her contemporaries exhibited both of these elements of aging with grace. Her actions were graceful. She was kind; she shared a warmth, lightness, and serenity with those who spent time with her. She was humble in her acceptance of the future yet honest about her fears and anxieties. She did not complain or burden others with her suffering. Sister Carline was also aging with grace in the form of the divine. Her days were filled with prayer and, in her words, "closeness with God." She embraced aging, and, as she grew older, she was held in God's embrace.

The goal of this chapter is to begin to understand this sense of grace and how the nuns cultivated it. I find that the grace, equanimity, and acceptance with which many of the nuns approached old age were cultivated through a lifetime of institutional practices informed by the theological notion of *kenosis*, the emptying out the self. In this chapter, I aim to show how habituated adherence to kenotic practices shaped the way the sisters experienced basic interactions with their material and social environment. This, in turn, contributed to their experiences of illness and death, thereby shaping their well-being at the end of life.

The grace and equanimity with which the sisters faced challenges, especially at the end of life, and the fulfillment they felt with their lives and community were cultivated through kenotic practices (practices of emptying out) that occurred at the macro- and microlevels. At the macrolevel were the large-scale institutional structures we have learned about, such as the convent administration and the three monastic vows of poverty, chastity, and obedience. At the microinteractional level, small-scale interactions such as the words the nuns spoke to each other and to the divine set the stage for the symbolic emptying out and filling up that is associated with kenosis and, ultimately, the equanimity they exhibited at the end of life.

This chapter explores these practices, including the nuns' three vows and how those vows were enacted in the nuns' lives and seemed to influence their aging experiences. My research will suggest that aging was experienced differently for those who adhered to the kenotic practices compared to those who did not. Vatican II and the specific ways that the Franciscan Sisters of the Sacred Heart handled the institutional changes played a major role in shaping how kenotic practices were introduced, incorporated, and embodied in the convent. As we have seen thus far, many of the rigorous institutional practices became optional for the nuns after Vatican II. In this period, the nuns were introduced to new institutional regulations and the nuns learned new ways to relate to the divine. As we saw in chapter 5, many sisters developed a more personalized, love-centered relationship with God. Some sisters continued to engage in strict institutional practices while others did not. The choices the sisters were allowed after Vatican II created a pronounced diversity in how kenosis was experienced in the convent. I suggest that this variation may correlate with some of the differences in well-being that I witnessed in the convent infirmary.

Kenosis: Emptying Out

Sister Carline, who we got to know in chapter 6, entered the Franciscan Sisters of the Sacred Heart Convent in 1943; she had just finished high school. When she joined, she and her peers entered a total institution that, to help her gain "freedom" from attachments to the material world, was designed to sever her ties with everything and everyone outside the convent. With her peers she took three vows: a vow of poverty, a vow of chastity, and a vow of obedience. The vow of poverty was designed to teach detachment to material things; the vow of chastity was designed to teach detachment from other humans; and the vow of obedience was meant to teach detachment from self-determination.

Poverty

When Sister Carline entered the convent, she, like the other young postulants was been given a list of items she could bring, including stockings and shoes in specific colors and styles. Every other possession had to be given up before she entered the convent gates. The nuns understood that the vow to live in poverty with minimal material possessions was designed to help them become closer to God. Following Saint Francis's rule, the nuns saw poverty as a virtue; attachment to material objects and money were potential distractions from a life of prayer and service.

The novitiate building in which the nuns lived was designed to encourage communality and, in doing so, denied the novices privacy. They shared sinks, showers, and bathrooms. They slept in twin beds in dorm rooms in which their personal space comprised only a small side table and a slim oak closet in which to hang their habits. As novices, the girls had to make formal requests to the novice mistress for any item they required—even small things like soap or toothpaste.

The vow of poverty became deeply ingrained in the nuns' everyday sense of morality. Sister Mary Bernard once told me a story about learning to navigate the vow of poverty as a young teacher. One day, she and a fellow sister received a grapefruit as a gift from a student. As she told me about the gift, she laughed, remembering with an intensity of emotion how difficult it was to discern what to do with the grapefruit. She recalled debating with the other sister whether it would be sinful to eat it or whether they must give it away as part of their obedience to the vow of poverty—and, if so, to whom. This story illustrates how internalized these structures were—not only structurally, through rules, but also emotionally. As the ninety-nine-year-old nun told me this story, I could see her continued struggle with the dual desires: wanting so much to be good and also yearning to taste that grapefruit, which she ultimately gave away.

Sister Mary Bernard's recollection of her struggle with the grapefruit shows how she had been retrained to attend to each moment of her life in a new way. The vow of poverty shaped the way she related to the gift, reframing the meaning she ascribed to it; she stopped seeing the gift as a fruit to be enjoyed and began to understand it as an indulgence that threatened to violate her vow of poverty. In light of her vows, the grapefruit had come to symbolize attachment to the world. It was one more thing that might threaten her attachment to the divine by shifting her attention away from God to worldly pleasure.

As we saw in chapter 6, early writings about monastic life positioned worldly pleasure as a hindrance to spiritual attainment. Church ideologies, especially in monastic settings, divided the world into the mundane and the spiritual. This division promoted the idea that attachments to the world reduced one's availability to the divine. The Ancrene Wisse, a monastic rule written for female anchorites in the thirteenth century, explicitly makes the argument that experiencing worldly pleasure precludes one from attaining spiritual pleasure in heaven (Millett 2009). One was expected to forgo all worldly pleasure in order to attain a place in heaven. In more contemporary monastic practice, evidence of the dichotomy between the spiritual and the worldly has endured. For example, Rebecca Lester (2005) has found that worldly attachments were framed as distractions that can prevent Mexican postulants from purifying the soul. In a twenty-first century context, material attachments are conceived of as distractions that can prevent nuns from experiencing the divine. Yet they were no longer held up as a something that could deny a sister access to heaven.

The training to live in poverty while avoiding material pleasure stayed with the nuns throughout their lives. In one conversation, Sister Rita described the recent death of Sister Pauline, a nun we had both known well. I had lived with Sister Pauline for a number of months in 2009 in the novitiate building. Sister Pauline had joined the convent in 1946 when she was sixteen years old and maintained many of the pre–Vatican II institutional practices more strictly than many of her peers. Sister Rita described Sister Pauline's adherence to the vow of poverty, even as she approached death:

When we were over there [at the hospital], we got talk about death, it came up in some way, and I said in passing, "Have you thought about dying?" And she said, "Oh, yeah, it comes and goes; just a thought, you know," but she said, "I don't think I'm quite ready."

When she got to the hospital, they did offer her the sacrament and she refused it; she said, "Oh, I'm just gonna have an angiogram done; that's not serious enough." I think Pauline by her very nature always weighed things as to whether or not I need this or not. Her life was very structured, and in that sense she led a very good, holy life. She was at a point, I think, in her life, where she was ready to meet God, that when they had to go to heart surgery, they told her the seriousness of it and the priest came and she said, "Yes, I'd like to be anointed," and she also said, "But if my heart stops, I do not wish to have resuscitation." So in the end she had made her choice, and there was her commitment and her willingness if life or death came to accept it.

Sister Rita interpreted her peer's refusal of the sacrament as a decision not to be wasteful in the most conservative sense. She never asked for more than what she absolutely needed. Sister Rita tells us that this reflected Sister Pauline's training and represents holiness and a moral good. This story shows how the vow of poverty could shape the way the nuns made significant life decisions.

Chastity

The second vow the nuns took was the vow of chastity, which prohibited not only sexual relations but restricted close attachments to any person. When the sisters entered the convent as novices, they were not allowed to return to their own homes and they were allowed to see their families only on chaperoned holiday visits. These rare family visits were highly regulated and took place on the convent grounds. Their letters home were limited and were read by the novice mistress, their direct superior. In addition, the nuns were not allowed to have what they called *particular friendships*, a term that referred to having a friend with whom one enjoyed spending time. If two novices seemed to be too close, they were separated. In their first few years in the convent, when the sisters were teenage girls who had just left their families, this often felt difficult as well as perplexing. Many nuns spoke to me about how surprising and painful it was to be separated from the new friends they had begun to get to know.

Sister Agnes Marie's description in chapter 1 of peeling potatoes in the convent kitchen while reciting ejaculations with the other postulants so that they would avoid chatting with each other exemplifies the institutional precautions against the development of friendships. The convent ban on "particular friendships" was part of a lifelong exercise meant to encourage spiritual discipline. This encouraged a shift away from attention to worldly relationships in favor of, in one nun's words, the "one true relationship; the relationship with the divine."

In an interview on National Public Radio, Catholic sister and social justice activist and author Sister Helen Prejean describes how the implementation of the vow of chastity had changed. Before Vatican II, she said, "we never talked about sexuality. Everything was sublimate, sublimate, sublimate, which means you just offered to God." After Vatican II, she describes an increased acceptance of the idea that sexuality was part of the natural human experience: "The challenge of celibacy is—it's not not to love anyone or not to love in friendship.

But you know that one of the levees around your river is that you will not go into full sexual expression with someone" (Prejean 2019). Many of the Franciscan Sisters of the Sacred Heart echoed the same idea that Prejean articulated: that sexuality is not inherently problematic. Instead, the vow reflects the fact that one consequence of sexual expression is that when people are sexually active, they become less open or able to devote themselves to loving all people. As Prejean explains, being sexually active is "so self-absorbing. And it closes you off because if you're in a sexual relationship with somebody, in that intimate a relationship, that's priority in your life. And you cannot simultaneously in your life be open to a whole lot of people. That's the challenge of celibacy, but not to live the shriveled-up life where you're not close to anybody" (Prejean 2019).

Through the vow of chastity, the nuns were encouraged to shift how they saw others. Rather than seeing others as individuals whom they might like or not like, relate to or not, they were encouraged to see all humans as if they were instantiations of the divine. Saint Augustine wrote that human friendship must be understood as way to relate to the divine, that in loving a friend one should be "loving the love of God in them." He added, "He truly loves a friend who loves God in the friend, either because God is actually present in the friend or in order that God may be so present" (Burt 1999, 62). In the convent, the vow of chastity was enacted through the process of "being God" to each other, a process in which the nuns learned to see others as an embodiment of the divine, treating others as they would treat Christ. For the nuns, "being God" or "being Christ" meant that they could model Jesus's behavior, acting in the world in the way they imagined Jesus would. It also meant that they would treat others as if those others embodied God, as if the they were interacting with Jesus himself.

In a talk on prayer that Sister Irma delivered to a group of retired nuns, she described the process of being Jesus to her peers (see also Corwin 2012b, 126):

EXAMPLE 1: BE THE LIGHT OF THE WORLD
Participants
SI: Sister Irma
SL: Sister Lupita
ALL: Group of nuns

01 SI: If Jesus says,
02   "Go out and be the light of the world,"
03   We are His presence.
04   The physical presence of Jesus among others,
05   and so, it is our vocation as Christians to be
06   that in some way.
07   Whether it's just praying for people,

```
08       or listening to people,
09       or serving people in any way,
10       but when we're in need,
11       we have to be gracious
12       to allow others to do that for us.
13       To share our pains,
14       to share our needs,
15       to let others listen to us,
16       so it's a two-way street.
17       If I am Jesus for Sister Lupita today,
18       tomorrow I may need Sister Lupita to be Jesus for
19       me.
20       Would you do that, Lupita?
21 ALL:  ((Laughter))
22 SL:   ((Nods))
23 SI:   She would do that.
24       All right.
```

In this passage, Sister Irma suggested that to be followers of Jesus, the sisters must not only serve others, but the sisters must accept help and "be gracious" when "we're in need" (lines 08–09). She says, "If I am Jesus for Sister Lupita today, tomorrow I may need Sister Lupita to be Jesus for me" (lines 15–16), a request that Sister Lupita consents to. In an interview, Sister Irma described to me the process of "being God" as one of her central goals. She said that she strives to "communicate the God in me with the God in them." One of the ways she did this was through the foot massages she regularly gave the other nuns. As she took the sisters' feet into her hands (see fig. 7.1), she embodied a position reminiscent to Jesus washing his disciples' feet, an image the sisters were all familiar with (see also Corwin 2012b).

The process of "being God" and envisioning God in another person was a kenotic practice. An example of sanctification through presence (as mentioned in chapter 1), it was a mode of interacting with others not as oneself or through the ego but as if the self were erased and filled with God. By imagining themselves as God—or as filled with God and imagining the person they were serving not as an individual whom they might like or not like, but as an embodiment of God—the sisters were enacting the vow of chastity.   ✝

Obedience

The third vow the nuns took, obedience, required that they unquestioningly obeyed their superiors. As Sister Genevieve, described obedience, "At the time I entered, what you were told was that you obeyed, you just did what you were told. You went where you were sent regardless of whether you liked it or not.

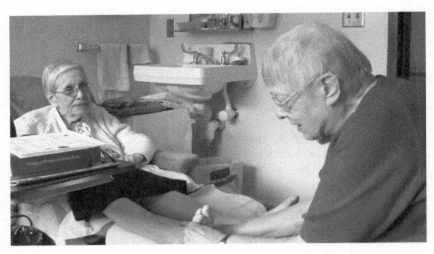

FIG. 7.1 Sister Irma "being God" as she massages a sister's feet. (Photo by the author)

Objections were pretty much forbidden." The vow of obedience was designed to encourage the sisters to relinquish the sense that they were in charge of their own lives or that they were their own self-determining agents. The theological goal of obedience, also a kenotic practice, was to teach the sisters to experience God as the ultimate authority. Their superiors, as church authorities, were seen as proxies with whom they could practice obedience to divine authority. The practice encouraged the sisters to be unattached to the details of their lives, such as where they lived, where they slept, and what they ate or wore, with the goal that nonattachment to worldly determination might help them cultivate a reliance on God alone.

To this end, the convent structured all of the material details of the nuns' days. As we learned in chapter 1, when the nuns entered the convent, the institution determined their daily schedules. As novices, they rose at 4:45 a.m. for prayers, for which they sat on hard benches. They worked, slept, and ate according to the time dictated by the convent bells. In the dining room they sat in rows, each with an identical plate of food, and ate in silence as a superior read prayers or spiritual texts. In an effort to train the novices in the practice of obedience, the convent authorities structured even the tiniest details of their lives. As we have seen, these practices aimed to shape each nun's material reality as a method to shape her internal reality. As Lester puts it, "obedience requires a woman to give up her own will, her claim to her own life" (2005, 74).

After the sisters took their vows (outlined in table 7.1) the Reverend Mother continued to determine most aspects of their lives, including their work. The sisters were sent to teach or serve in parishes across the region, and these assignments could change at a moment's notice. Each summer the sisters

Table 7.1
Vows: Meaning and implementation

Vow	Meaning	Implementation: Emptying Out	Implementation: Filling Up
Poverty	Detachment from material things	Stripped of material things	Helps focus on spiritual pursuits and meaning
Chastity	Detachment from people	Stripped of connection with others (letters, visits, personal friendships)	The divine becomes the primary loving relationship
Obedience	Detachment from self-determination	Stripped of freedom of movement, freedom of choice	Actions are seen as inspired by the divine

packed all of their belongings into a trunk and returned to the motherhouse for a summer retreat and convent-wide meetings. At these yearly meetings each received a small white slip of paper called an *obedience* on which her work assignment for the following year was written. They had to ready themselves for any possible assignment. Before the summer, as they packed up, they had to say goodbye to everyone they had known—their fellow teachers, parishioners, or students—in case they did not return. A sister could be teaching at a school for twenty-five years of her life in one place and then receive an obedience informing her that her next assignment was to work in the kitchen at the motherhouse or fly across the world to work as a missionary. The nuns sometimes felt that the work assignments, in one sister's words, "did not have any relation to their abilities." Nevertheless, they were required to follow them.

The sisters were required to be obedient to their superiors in matters both major and minor. One of the sisters described her first meal in the convent. She, like all the sisters, was served a glass of milk with her meal. She was allergic to milk and did not drink it. The novice mistress insisted she drink the milk even though she claimed to be allergic. The novice drank it and later threw up. While she was not required to drink milk again, the interaction nevertheless served to demonstrate to the novice that she was no longer in charge of her own body and actions. The superiors—and, symbolically, the divine—were in charge of the novices' actions, determining what they ate and drank, how they spent their time, and how they related to others. The nuns were being taught to think of their lives as determined not by themselves but by the divine.

These strict institutional practices rendered the convent a *total institution*—what Erving Goffman (1961) has described as designed to disrupt the self-determination, autonomy, and freedom of those within it. When a person enters a total institution, such as a convent, asylum, or prison, she is stripped of symbols of the self and identity. The nuns, for example, were assigned new names, new clothes, and new rules by which to live. They dressed in white gowns symbolizing wedding dresses to take the vows that sealed their union with Christ. Goffman considers this process a "curtailment of the self" whereby the nuns were stripped of their identity and individual personhood: "The admission process can be characterized as a leaving off and a taking on, with the midpoint marked by physical nakedness. Leaving off of course entails a dispossession of property, important because persons invest self-feelings in their possessions. Perhaps the most significant of these possessions is not physical at all, loss of one's full name can be a great curtailment of the self" (1961, 18). Goffman's "curtailment of the self" is perfectly aligned with the theological goals of kenosis, whereby the convent stripped the nuns of their identity so that they might be filled with God.

When they took their vows, the nuns prostrated themselves on the floor, ritually enacting a symbolic death from the world. Once in the convent, these institutional practices helped shape a new identity and experience. Unlike prisons and asylums, the monastic total institution was designed with the goal of moral and spiritual transformation. Michel Foucault argues that Christianity, which involves the ideology of salvation, holds that through a transformation of the self an individual can move from one reality to another, "from death to life, from time to eternity" (1988, 43). As we have seen, Christian monastic ideals maintain that this process can achieve a "purification of the soul."

Foucault discusses the process through which a monastic submits complete control in obedience as a "sacrifice of the self" through which the individual develops a new "technology of the self" (Foucault 1988, 45). While Goffman's description of the total institution focuses on the role of the institution in shaping individual experience, Foucault, in his discussion of the development of technologies of the self, focuses on how the individual "acts on himself" within particular institutional and ideological settings (1988, 18). While both the institutional role and the actions of the individual within the institution were central to the nuns' stories before Vatican II, in the time following Vatican II, when convent regulations loosened up, much of the work of obedience was self-imposed by sisters striving to transform themselves.

In both time periods, surveillance played an important role in the regimentation afforded by the convent as a total institution. In the convent the nuns did not have private space, and their daily activities occurred in the company of their peers. For instance, figure 7.2 depicts the shared bathrooms in the novitiate building.

Surveillance was within the purview not only of convent authorities but also of other sisters who were involved in a shared spiritual and moral

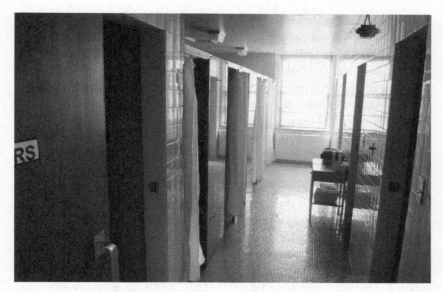

FIG. 7.2 Shared showers. (Photo by the author)

self-making project. This constant surveillance restricted the nuns' social mobility and flexibility, forcing them to see themselves through an institutional gaze. As Goffman writes, the surveillance of others makes a person's infraction, whether against authoritative codes, "likely to stand out in relief against the visible, constantly examined compliance of others" (1961, 7). In addition, once the sisters joined the convent, their infractions were no longer seen as individual behavior. The nuns were now representations of the institution itself and responsible not only for themselves but also for the Church's spiritual and moral well-being.

Kenosis

In what sounds to an outsider like a paradox, the vow of obedience was designed to create internal or spiritual freedom through the structured disavowal of external freedom, individuation, and self-determination. The discomfort involved in giving up individuation and self-determination were seen as a necessary step in the path toward sanctification and unification with the divine. These processes were based largely in the theological premise of kenosis.

The term *kenosis*, derived from the Greek for "emptiness," first appears in Philippians 2:1–11, where Christ is said to have "emptied [*ekenōsen*] himself, taking the form of a servant." Kenosis is translated variously as emptying oneself, a death of the self, making oneself nothing, and a "voluntary decentering of the self" (Westphal 2005, 22). In this context, emptying the self or ego allows a person to make room for the divine. This notion of emptiness is often interpreted as selfless action, engaging with the world selflessly. Kenosis can be variously interpreted as "being a person for others, loving, giving oneself, letting go" (Cronin 1992, 7). Kenosis is also associated with humility and the process of letting go of individuality—precisely what the nuns' vows were designed to do. Although in some contexts kenosis might seem like a choice, as in the "voluntary decentering of the self" quoted above, it is perhaps more accurately interpreted as an attitude. While one cannot determine what happens in life, a kenotic attitude, in which one rids the self of attachments, can shape how one experiences even traumatic life events. Renée van Riessen, a philosopher of Christianity, describes a story by J. M. Coetzee as an example of kenosis. While the story never mentions the term itself, Van Riessen has argued that it is as an exemplar of kenosis. In the story, which offers insight into the notion of kenosis in its various interpretations, two characters give up the things that have built their identity and bring them joy.

In Coetzee's story, a university professor is accused by a student of abuse of power and position. The professor is forced to leave his job at a university to live with his daughter on a farm. During his stay, the farm is plundered by a group of men who rape the adult daughter, Lucie, who becomes pregnant. Coatzee describes Lucie as turning inward as she "lets everything take its course." Lucie gives up her independent life to raise her daughter. As Van Riessen notes, "Lucie's attitude is a mixture of resignation and perseverance: she is willing to give up who she is (an independent woman with her own business) in order to stay in the place where she loves to be, on her own land, with the animals and plants dear to her" (2007, 175). In the story, Lucie lets go of her independence, her business, and even her physical body and sense of anger following physical violence.

Van Riessen interprets this as a kenotic story, writing, "It's always about letting go, letting go of the past, of an influential position at the university; letting go of a successful future that would seem the natural destiny for the daughter of a professor. Letting go of positions of power and the status connected with them" (2007, 175). It is also about accepting the difficult or painful events in life that cannot be changed. In Van Riessen's interpretation of the story, Lucie's acceptance of her child and her role as a mother following the brutal act of violence is a kenotic act. She grieves the tragedy that has occurred, but she ultimately accepts what has happened and moves forward to accept her life as it now stands. However brutally, her life has been transformed, and she accepts her new state.

Although the story does not concern an attachment to the sacred, a key component in the nuns' understanding of kenosis, it is nonetheless useful in understanding the concept. The story conveys the sense that kenosis is not easy and does not protect one from life's tragedies. It does not allow a person to avoid the world, but rather to accept life as it comes—good and bad—and move forward. The goal of kenosis is not to avoid life and its tragic or joyous events (an impossible feat) but to train the mind and body to react to these events evenly and with acceptance.

The process of emptying oneself of the outside world and filling oneself with God has been incorporated into contemporary Western ideologies. The Alcoholics Anonymous command, "Let go and let God" is also an example of kenosis in practice. The concept of emptying the self involves moving aside the ego or the self and allowing oneself to move forward, accepting whatever comes in life with equanimity.

Catholic interpretations of kenosis are distinct from secular interpretations (such as Coatzee's story) in that they emphasize an ultimate "filling up" with God. Catholics see this process as making space within that can then be filled up with divine love. Through their vows and institutional practices, nuns empty themselves of material, social, and internal connections while simultaneously developing a deep spiritual sense of divine connection and love. This emptiness is seen as creating a space in which "the sacred can incarnate itself in bodily being and behavior" (Benson and Wirzba 2005a, 5).

For Christians, the ultimate kenotic act was God, in human form as Jesus, emptying himself to become "a slave" (Mensch 2005, 65). Saint Francis, the founder of the Franciscan order, for example, focused on the kenosis of Jesus Christ, who emptied himself of his own divinity in order to take on the nature of a human and ultimately accept his death by crucifixion. As Kevin Cronin notes, "This humbling, this emptying, this letting go was something Francis longed for in imitation of his love, Jesus Christ" (1992, 2).

Buddhism shares the concept that emptiness is key to the path that allows individuals to approach enlightenment. In Buddhist teachings, this path toward enlightenment and freedom from suffering involves the cultivation of nonattachment, the practice of emptying oneself of attachment to the world, a process that requires an acceptance of the transience of all things. The theme of emptiness occurs in Hinduism as well. Sarah Lamb describes a resonant process among Hindu practitioners in West Bengal, India. By way of example, Lamb describes marriage, a time when young girls are forced to relinquish their ties to their natal home: "The bride's surname and patrilineal membership would also be formally changed to those of her husband. In this way, her marriage was generally interpreted as obscuring and greatly reducing, although not obliterating, the connections she once enjoyed with her natal home. . . . For a girl, then, preparing to marry was like a first confrontation with Mortality" (1997, 291). This symbolic death is not unlike that of nuns who, upon entering the convent, have to give up connections to their families and the world outside the convent.

Lamb describes the local concept of *maya*, which she translates as attachment, affection, compassion, or love. She writes that in Mangaldihi, West

Bengal, people saw themselves as connected to the "persons, places, and things with which they lived and interacted." She describes the ties, or *maya*, as increasing over a lifetime. She writes that elderly persons find themselves in what she describes as a "paradox" in older age; when in anticipating leaving the world and separating from the people, places, and things they know, they experience these ties as the strongest (1997, 283, 285). As Lamb notes,

> The greatest problem of *maya* in old age is that of how people will free their souls when they die. Maya, according to people in Mangaldihi, can quite literally "bind" a person (or the person's soul, *atma*) to his or her body, habitat, and relationships, caught as in a "net" (*jal*), and thereby unable to die, even if very ill and decrepit, and unable to depart from his or her previous habitat and relations after death. Not only can *maya* or attachments cause people to hang on in this way in a state of decrepitude without dying, but *maya* can also make the process of dying itself very slow and painful. (1997, 289)

Elder Hindus in West Bengal thus find themselves engaged in a process of methodically cutting their ties with the world. Lamb describes elderly widows and men avoiding particular foods that might excite worldly passions or attachments and dressing in white, a color regarded as "cooling." Elderly women and men also engage in celibacy and antisocial activities such as cursing or arguing, which she describes as "techniques of self-alienation." She adds, "People diminished their ties of *maya* to things as well, by emptying themselves of their favorite possessions in late life—giving away property, jewelry, favorite saris, keepsakes. All of the techniques of decentering, cooling, and emptying mentioned above were felt in Mangaldihi to be effective methods for shrinking those personal extensions that are known as *maya*" (1997, 289).

The kenotic theme of emptying oneself of ties to the material and social world appears in a number of cultural contexts with some variations. Lamb's work in West Bengal, for example, shows that for elderly Hindus, it serves to help individuals transition into the end of life and into death. Kenosis as experienced by Catholic nuns involves both letting go of attachments and "filling up" through a concentrated relationship with God.

Filling Up

Thomas Merton, the renowned Trappist monk and author, writes, "Detachment from things does not mean setting up a contradiction between 'things' and 'God' . . . as if [God's] creatures were His rivals. We do not detach ourselves from things in order to attach ourselves to God, but rather we become detached from ourselves in order to see and use all things in and for God" (1961, 21).

Philosopher Emmanuel Levinas considers the letting go of oneself involved in kenosis to be a "devotion" and "act of dedication" to the divine. Similarly, Van Riessen considered what she named the "humiliation" involved in the defacement of the self to be an articulation "of God's transcendence" (2007, 179). In this context, kenosis involves detachment from the self with the explicit goal of coming closer to the divine.

In my conversations with Sister Carline when she was dying, she told me about her experience filling up with God. She described an inner life that, in her view, kept her buoyant throughout the cancers and continued to buoy her in the face of death. She spent the majority of her time meditating on Christ the child, thinking to herself about "how much He must have loved us" to come to earth. She was in awe that, in her words, "of all the places in the infinite universe He could go, He chose to come to us, to our tiny planet." A sense of wonder and joy overtook her as she described the sense of love she attributed to this act.

From both her bed and her reclining chair, Sister Carline could rest her eyes on a small figurine depicting the infant Jesus in the manger on one of her shelves. With her eyes on the crèche, she regularly meditated on "God's love for us, as humans." Following this meditation, she described "traveling" across the wall, moving her eyes eight feet to the right, where a San Damiano Cross hung. With her eyes resting on Jesus on the cross, she would meditate on the idea that "God loved us so much that he was willing to live as a human and to suffer for us, out of love." She emphasized the idea that his death on the cross was a form of compassion, saying that "suffering is love."

Like many of the nuns, Sister Carline's prayers centered on communion with God. As we saw in chapter 6, she said she prayed for spiritual healing, which she understood to be a closeness with God, a "healing of the soul." When speaking about that healing of the soul, Sister Carline told me about a retreat that she had taken a few decades earlier, her first retreat led by a spiritual director. She said that her personal focus for the retreat was first to become closer with God and second to address a fear she had been experiencing at the time, one she described as irrational but very powerful. She did not tell me what it was that she feared, just that she wanted to be free from it. When she told the spiritual director about this desire, the director suggested that Sister Carline embrace the fear and accept it. She reported that later in the retreat, she experienced a powerful vision; a crystal goblet inside of which was a teardrop. She described the teardrop as "adorable" and "loveable," with big eyes blinking at her. She said that she opened up her arms to embrace the teardrop and it jumped into her arms and dissolved into her.

Sister Carline explained that to her the teardrop represented her fear. The embrace brought forth a novel feeling of being able to love and accept this fear.

The goblet, she said, represented God. Each beveled edge represented a different facet of God such that "you could never see them all at once." Sister Carline said that in the vision the teardrop also represented her body, and her body represented Jesus. She said she experienced Jesus loving her and wrapping his arms around her in an embrace echoing the one she gave the teardrop.

Sister Carline explained that this vision seemed to her simultaneously crazy and very real. She said she knew it was real because it had a tangible effect on her mind and body. Her fear was completely gone from that day on. Sister Carline said that in the many years since that retreat, she revisited and meditated on this vision as a part of her daily prayers. In these prayers, God embraced her as she dissolved into him.

Like Sister Carline, many of the nuns suffering from chronic conditions did not focus on their own pain but, drawing on years of kenotic training, focused their attention away from it and let it rest on the divine. These women seemed to experience a remarkable sense of calm and what Sister Carline called an "abiding love" even as they faced physical pain and suffering at the end of life. This skill—refocusing attention away from pain or mental anguish onto feelings of divine love, peace, and calm—seemed to be bolstered by the kenotic practices they engaged both before and after Vatican II.

Early in their lives, pre–Vatican II institutional training forced the nuns to learn to shed attachments to material things, to families and friends, and to the ego and desire for self-determination. After Vatican II many nuns began to practice embodied forms of prayer in which they cultivated a personalized relationship with the divine and an experience of divine presence, as we saw in chapter 5. They experienced the divine not only through verbal interaction such as spoken prayer but also through divine presence, a presence they experienced sometimes physically, as a feeling, a hand in theirs, or as a generalized sense of divine peace, calm, or love.[1] We saw that this process was an ongoing struggle for Sister Carline in chapter 6. "I've been praying especially for that inner peace that I can accept whatever God's will is," she told me. "I kept praying and I kept praying it, and, sometimes I'd be just, you know, kind of, not . . . not resisting but kind of struggling with it. And so as time has been going on, I do feel more peace with where I am, knowing that I feel like God's peace has been given to me and, and I'm praying that it even goes deeper, that it just keeps going. I don't want to be struggling. I want to, I want to welcome death." Yet, even as she struggled, she came to have the tools to approach her own death with strength and peace.

Many of the nuns who adhered to kenotic practices seemed to accept physical change with remarkable equanimity. Sister Mary Bernard, who fretted over whether the vow of poverty forbid her from accepting the grapefruit, exemplified this sense of peace in the face of major change. At age ninety-nine, she had been in the convent for eighty-three years. Even after the changes following

Vatican II, Sister Mary Bernard strictly adhered to the kenotic practices of poverty, chastity, and obedience as they had been taught to her in her youth. In one conversation, for example, she spoke to me about material attachments. She told me that when she died, she would prefer to own absolutely nothing. Although she was not ill at the time, she told me that she was continually trying to give away everything she owned, including small trinkets, figurines, or books individuals had given her over the years, as well as one small side table.

Sister Mary Bernard reported to me that when one sister had died, the community put the deceased sister's things in a room and other sisters had the opportunity to stop by the room to take items they wanted. She reported that the entire room was taken up by the possessions that had belonged to the single sister. Sister Mary Bernard was dismayed, reporting this incident as an example of extreme excess and deviance from the vow of poverty. She wanted to meet death in complete poverty, owning nothing at all, and also requested that her body be cremated because the cemetery was filling up. She suggested that cremation would save the "fuss" and leave space for others to be buried in the future.

Each time I visited Sister Mary Bernard, she would tell me that one must "accept what God gives you." During the summer that I was pregnant with my son, she told me often that she prayed that my baby would be healthy and that the delivery would go well. She then added, "but you have to accept what God gives you. The hardest thing is to accept the difficult things, but you know He loves you most with those because he's asking you to go through that for Him." I felt that she was continually preparing me to accept the possibility of loss in case the pregnancy and birth did not go well.

I witnessed Sister Mary Bernard go through one of these "difficult things." Although she lived in the infirmary where she had access to nursing assistance if she needed it, she still lived an active life. She would fly through the motherhouse, visiting with her neighbors, traveling downstairs to Mass and to the dining hall at least three times a day. I often saw her tiny frame whiz by on her way to pick up spiritual books in the reading room or to visit with a friend. Despite her activity, Sister Mary Bernard had limited circulation in her left leg, and a doctor told her that she would have to have it amputated above the knee. Before the operation, she told me that she did not know how she would live without her leg. She seemed fearful of life with only one leg, but repeated what I had heard her say many times, that "you have to accept what God gives you." Marveling that she would continue to live at age ninety-eight with the only one leg, she said, "God must have more work for me to do on this planet."

Following the amputation and recovery, Sister Mary Bernard was almost as social and energetic as before. She often positioned her wheelchair in the hallway where she could chat with whoever passed by. She told me that although she had thought she would not be able to live without her leg, she simply accepted what God had given her. She told me that her faith carried her through the operation and continued to buoy her up. "I know that God is good to me," she explained.

It seems that sisters like Sister Mary Bernard who practiced acceptance and obedience throughout their lives seemed to have an ability to draw on this practice in the face of major life changes like the loss of a limb. She met her operation with optimism and a determination to accept God's will (and the doctor's orders) with obedience and grace. She interpreted the challenge as evidence of divine love, and she seemed to come out of the experience with remarkable equanimity.

An Erosion of Kenotic Practices

In the late 1960s and the decades following Vatican II, the institutional structures that enforced kenotic practices gave way to individual freedoms meant to allow individuals to commune with the divine in more personal ways. Nuns in many convents gained freedoms they had not previously had, such as the ability to choose how they dressed, to develop and maintain close relationships with friends and family, to choose where they worked and lived, and to pray independently. Many of the sisters I met welcomed these changes, as they felt they that the new freedoms allowed them to deepen their spirituality, to get to know God on their own terms, and to better serve those in need.

The nuns still took the three vows of poverty, chastity, and obedience, but the meanings of the vows changed. Instead of emphasizing material poverty, the nuns emphasized a poverty of the soul. They were now allowed to have material possessions, and the vow of poverty thus became a metaphorical emphasis on an internal state. As one nun articulated, "The idea of poverty is not so much that you get permission for everything you use but of living simply, and being responsible. It's now more about the responsible use of goods."

Obedience also shifted to mean an obedience to the divine or to a "God within" rather than an institutional power. This meant that the sisters had much more input in determining the details of their days. The nuns became free to determine their places of work, where they lived, and many other details of their lives. While the convent maintained some rules, obedience became more personally conceived as each nun focused on her own understanding of God's will.

The vow of chastity changed as well. There was no longer a ban on particular friendships. Echoing Sister Helen Prejean, one the nuns described the vow of chastity: "For me it means that it's a matter of responsible use of one's sexual energies, that it's more than just that you don't get married or that don't have sex. That you don't, that your love is much broader than that, it's a love for all people. And it makes you freer. The vow of celibacy is kind of freeing to demonstrate your love for all."

For many of the nuns who had lived for decades in the convent before the changes of Vatican II were implemented, these changes did not radically alter their relationship with the material world. Sister Carline, for instance, who no longer donned a habit and was able to choose her work and determine her prayer practices, continued to live in small convents and never acquired many material things. She continued to practice the fundamental kenotic rituals of emptying the self and filling herself with the divine.

Some of the nuns were more impacted by Vatican II than others. While their peers maintained many of the practices they had developed before Vatican II, some sisters took advantage of institutional changes more dramatically. For example, Sister Marie,[2] who had joined the convent in the 1940s, was trained under the same rigor as Sister Carline, but when Vatican II introduced increasing freedom to the nuns' lives, Sister Marie embraced them. She took a job teaching in a city where there was no community convent. She lived alone in an apartment. Community members gave her gifts: beautiful figurines, sculptures of angels, and shelving units to hold these treasures. She developed deep and loving relationships with a large community, ties that were evidenced in her apartment: framed photographs of herself with dear friends, Christmas cards, loving statements. She was an important community figure, garnering praise and support for her work. She had shelves of books, both spiritual and secular, and even newspaper clippings noting her good works.

When Sister Marie began having trouble walking and struggling to keep up with her job, she resisted suggestions from convent authorities that she return to the motherhouse where caregivers could help her in the convent's assisted living wing. The idea of giving up her apartment and returning to shared housing pained her; she did not want to lose her freedom. Finally, Sister Marie fell and broke her hip. It was only after the injury that she moved to the motherhouse.

In my field notes in July 2010, I wrote about an encounter with Sister Marie and my own initial comparison between her and Sister Carline:

> Today, I had a brief visit with Sister Marie, who is now home from the hospital again. She was lying in bed, covered in a sheet, on her side. She looked miserable. She turned toward me. One of the first things she said was how upset she was that she will miss Jubilee. This strikes me as so different from many of the other nuns like Sister Carline, who, when she had to miss Easter with her family, seems to handle disappointment with such grace. She kept her optimism up through her prayers for acceptance, and surrender. Sister Marie, on the other hand, is so caught up in a different type of prayer: prayer for her own healing that she just clings to health, what she's missing out on.

The congregational minister, the head nurse, and many of the sisters spoke to me about the phenomenon of sisters who resisted retirement. They described this as a new development that had emerged in recent decades. They each said that that many of the older nuns were struggling with retirement and enduring emotional strife as they had to give up their freedoms. The head nurse, who had worked in the convent infirmary for decades, said, "Comforts such as independent living have made the sisters much more attached to their things, their individual space—for example, having their own bathroom." She noted that this attachment caused strife for the sisters as they grew older and had to transition into smaller rooms, leave their jobs and apartments, and give up their things.

In the quality of life questionnaire I administered, Sister Marie, like her peers, reported that her life was highly meaningful, purposeful, and worthwhile and that she felt "completely" cared for and supported. Yet she reported that she was slightly more afraid of the future than her peers and reported just slightly higher experiences of depression and anxiety on the questionnaire. Significantly, however, her assessment of her overall physical, spiritual, and mental quality of life was extremely low, far below the majority of her peers. In my extensive interviews with her and other nuns like her, it became clear that Sister Marie and some others experienced daily emotional strife as they anticipated losing their independence. She resented suggestions that she could no longer live independently, even though she relied on a number of her peers to help her with daily tasks.

Unlike the strictly regimented practices before Vatican II, the kenotic practices that emerged after Vatican II were usually voluntary. For example, as was discussed in chapter 4, the sisters in later decades have been asked to be involved in planning their own funerals. The process required that the nuns address their own mortality. I see this as a kenotic act that, although voluntary, encouraged the sisters to face the inevitability of death.

Sister Rita described the process of planning her own funeral:

I think as you age you also change your view of death. I did it then [the first time] thinking that it was sort of ritual, this is what I would like, it was really personal, but then, one of the persons who I had to carry my cross died on me, so, you know, it's like people changed, they're no longer part of your life in some way, so this time I did it about six months ago and really took time to pray, to look at readings, to look at where I am, what really appeals to me, who I would like to have part of it. For me the funeral represents who I am when I was here, and I'd like them to remember good things about me and some funny things, and if there were some of my faults, yes, those too, you know; I think that all that can be worked into a homily.

As she described the planning process, she also described her expectations for what death was and should be, and how people should approach their own and others' deaths:

> I would like you to come and I don't want you sit around and mope and cry and if you cry tears fine but I don't think funerals have to be, they're a celebration, because death is simply the step over the line, its passing on. . . . That's what we do, we pass on. . . . We begin dying at birth and the process is slowly takes, we go through the stages of life, and why not then be, we come to the threshold and the stepping over is what we have to do. Right now in my life I feel comfortable with that. And I think maybe planning the funeral solidified that for, that it's—it's made me less fearful. I think for me the fear is in, Will there be pain in the dying? And I think that's true for a lot of people.

Sister Rita said that as she planned her funeral, she became less fearful of her own death and began to accept the inevitability of it.

This story is not, however, a simple narrative that pre–Vatican II practices promote well-being. It is not possible to speak to those who lived their whole lives under Vatican II, but I did hear from those who knew them. This second-hand evidence combined with the historical data from chapters 5 and 6 on conceptions of authority, God, and pain before Vatican II suggests that those who lived and died before Vatican II did not necessarily benefit from a greater sense of peace and well-being. Sister Laura, who spent time with her older peers in the infirmary, describes the end of life before Vatican II as often difficult:

> People [were] very, very fearful about not doing the rule, not doing exactly what [they] have to do. . . . I think that was part of the old structure of religious life, where we were so structured and so conformed and fearful because we were afraid that if we didn't do this, we would be sent home and . . . that, you know, you think you don't do good you're bound to hell. I can think of a couple of sisters who needed to be comforted and they needed to be reassured. Not just—not by me, but by a priest. . . . The fear of the Lord, even though it's in the Bible, isn't the kind of fear that's going to put you into hell.

Sister Laura's description of fear describes pre–Vatican II sentiments similar to those Sister Rita described in chapter 5. As we saw in that chapter, the conception of an authoritarian, punitive God changed after Vatican II as the nuns developed a relationship with the divine that emphasized love and compassion.

In the years that I have known the Franciscan Sisters of the Sacred Heart, I have met many nuns like Sister Rita and Sister Carline who continued most of the kenotic practices they had engaged in before Vatican II. They collected few personal items, continued to share space and chores with others in communal convent housing, and accepted the limitations of their bodies with relative grace as they retired from work and entered the assisted living or infirmary wings of the convent. I also encountered a number of nuns like Sister Marie who enjoyed the freedoms associated with Vatican II, accrued many material things, lived independently, and became attached to the people and places where they worked. Like Sister Marie, many of these nuns struggled with depression and inner anguish as they mourned the loss of independence as they grew older and developed chronic conditions.

The peace and acceptance that nuns like Sister Carline demonstrated seem to be most robust in nuns who were trained under Vatican II and who maintained the kenotic practices even after the convent no longer enforced them and who also have devoted much of their lives to "filling up" with a loving God. It seems that the unique combination of pre–Vatican II institutionalized disengagement from material, social, and personal attachments, along with a less fearful and more loving relationship with God after Vatican II, was a powerful aid to those at the end of life.

Summary: Kenosis and Acceptance

Kenotic practices can be seen as a skill that can be honed over a lifetime. As with any skill, there is variation in how easily it is picked up, practiced, maintained, and mastered. For those who practice it, it may be a key factor in contributing to psychological and spiritual well-being at the end of life. Research has shown that individuals can train themselves to experience the world in particular ways. Through habituated practices, individuals come to shape the ways in which they experience their bodies and the world. For example, through prayer, evangelical Christians train themselves to attend to the world and sensory input in ways that allow them to experience God more frequently and with more immediacy (Luhrmann 2012; Luhrmann, Nusbaum, and Thisted 2010).

Habituated institutional practices can influence individuals' experiences of aging and the end of life. The kenotic training in which the nuns engaged primed them to attend to the experiences of "attachment" in particular ways. When they were young, the nuns were required to let go of feelings of attachment to loved ones and friends and to concentrate their feelings of love and attachment on the divine. When they were asked to give up work they loved or possessions they enjoyed, they experienced the process of letting go as an extension of their love of the divine and their compassion for humankind.

Through these habituated practices the nuns seemed to have trained themselves to respond to the inevitable losses that come with aging in the world (such as an amputated leg, cancer, or death) with equanimity, acceptance, and relative peace. When the nuns were required to give up mobility or comfort as their bodies gave out in old age, they engaged in the same pattern, redirecting their attention from the things they were giving up to focus on God's love.

Conclusion

· ·

Eight years after my first trip to the Franciscan Sisters of the Sacred Heart Convent, I rose at 6:30 one morning, kissed my children goodbye to leave my home to return to the sisters. My son rolled over in bed and said, "I'm too emotional to say goodbye" and went back to sleep. My daughter clung to me. When I pried her off, she waved from the front door as I pulled out of our driveway in the East Bay of California to drive to the airport. Eight hours later, I got off the plane, stepped outside into the deep embrace of the humid Midwest summer. In a rental car I drove the hour and a half from the airport to the convent. The landscape once again struck me with its marvel of greens. On the car stereo, I struggled to find National Public Radio, and, failing, landed on a Christian rock station, where I listened to men sing pop songs of praise and tenderness. The moon was full and heavy in the sky, a milky balloon. I passed cows, billboards, and the occasional car lot. I felt full of trepidation. I'd left my children, my home, the relative comfort of the dry California heat. Why do I keep coming back? I wondered. Despite the time I had spent in the convent and my many trips back, fear knotted in my belly, anticipating feeling alone or foreign. So many of the women I had known had died. What, I thought to myself as the young man on the radio crooned about Christ's love, am I doing here?

As I turned the corner at the gas station to enter town, I could see the brick convent wall that once symbolically and physically kept the sisters from the outside world. The iron gates were propped permanently open. The moon beamed its light over the convent grounds. The heat enveloped me in the smell of soil, worms, and mowed grass. I realized, looking over the blinking landscape, that fireflies were dancing across the lawn. I calmed a little, taking in the beauty of a Midwestern summer.

Sister Paula had waited up for me to let me into the novitiate building and greeted me with a smile. Although nothing had changed since my many previous visits, she kindly, tediously showed me how the key worked, how to make coffee, reminded me where the chapel was. She told me that another sister had died on Thursday, someone with whom I had played cards with every Monday and Wednesday night during previous stays at the convent.

Sister Paula paused after giving me this news to ask what brought me here this time. I told her that I had been thinking about presence, the presence of the divine, and was hoping to talk to people about their experiences. Suddenly she lit up. She stopped her slow uneven walk down the hallway and looked at me beaming. "Ooh, honey," she said, "you'll have some great conversations." Facing me in the hallway, her blue eyes beamed as she told me about her sense that when people die their spirit remains with us. That they are never gone. That they move from life to transformed life.

I thought, This is why I keep coming back. There is something ineffable about the love and joy that these women have spent their lives cultivating. The sparkle in Sister Paula's eyes as she spoke with me about her peer, our friend, who had died is precisely where the heart of this story lies. The most important piece of the nuns' story is not the quantitative measures of well-being, nor is it the nuns' record of health or longevity. To live a long life, or to avoid heart disease longer than one's contemporaries: these are remarkable feats that surely keep epidemiologists busy crunching data and theorizing about causal mechanisms. But, for me, the anthropologist who has spent the past decade living with, visiting, and thinking about these women, what keeps me writing and thinking about them is the sparkle in Sister Paula's eyes as she tells me about our dear friend's death. This woman in her eighties with pronounced arthritis who had spent time in and out of the infirmary, had waited up until late into the night to show me to a room I knew well and had stayed in many times before. More profound to me than the medical achievements is this: being old, being in pain, and still sparkling with joy and driven to service.

The Franciscan Sisters of the Sacred Heart live in a community built on interdependence, shared spirituality, and an acceptance of decline and death. This book has aimed to show that these ideals—community, interdependence, and meaningful decline—reveal themselves in microinteractional moments. They are values that manifest in the nuns' everyday lives as they stay up late to explain to an anthropologist friend of the community how the coffeemaker works, as they pray for the grace to "accept what comes," or as they coordinate a game of cards with a sister who in old age can no longer speak or move as she once did. These practices, just like the prayers that socialize sisters into particular ways of aging, are simple actions that together shape the nuns' experiences at the end of life. In a society where scientific findings are often translated into seemingly quick fixes, as in "Eating blueberries every day improves heart health"

(University of East Anglia, 2019), ethnographies provide a different lesson. Rather than isolating single threads that might explain social phenomena or health outcomes, anthropological inquiry reveals how interconnected cultural values and ideals are with the habitual practices—the small acts—we engage in.

One of the motivations for you as a reader to pick up this book may have been to think through how you, too, might age "well." The Franciscan Sisters of the Sacred Heart are deeply embedded in North American culture. They live in the United States, are practicing Christians, and are remarkably productive members of society. Yet their transition into old age takes a very different course than that of most Americans.

I recently ran a small research study in a retirement community near my home in California. I could not have found myself in a context that embraced the successful aging paradigm more. The community is mostly middle or upper middle class. The men and women in my study were remarkably active, many of them biking or walking many miles each week. Every individual had an active social life and a full social calendar. Much as Sarah Lamb found with the elders she worked with in Boston (2014), many of the men and women at the beginning of our work together articulated that the effects of aging could be avoided or delayed by staying active and fit, eating well, and keeping themselves engaged. And yet, as conversations grew deeper, these active, healthy older adults revealed a deep emotional struggle as they spoke about feeling lonely, invisible, irrelevant to the rest of society, and fearful of the impending specter of their own and others' decline and deaths.

Discrete healthy aging tactics such as eating well and staying active certainly can be attractive to those hoping to maintain health and well-being. Even if they work, however, they only push decline and death farther down the road. Ultimately, everyone who lives long enough must encounter decline and the end of life. What the nuns' stories demonstrate is that in a society that continues to stigmatize aging, aging well involves more than adopting a simple set of behaviors (like "eating well"). Sister Paula's eyes sparkled as she walked down the hall with me, wobbling to accommodate the arthritis in her knees, not because her community has outsmarted or avoided aging. Her eyes shone with joy despite the late hour, despite the death of her friends, and despite the pain of her arthritis because her life and community were filled with cultural practices that supported her as she aged. For Sister Paula, being in the presence of others and the presence of God was more important than being productive. She had tools, developed over a lifetime, that help her to accept her own decline with grace. She held the knowledge that decline and change were essential, natural, elements of life. She knew that as she grew older and declined, she would continue to be valued, held by her community, and thanked for her prayers.

While I have tried to make clear that the nuns' experiences of aging are intertwined with their specific cultural and historical practices, there are nevertheless some lessons we can take with us.

Lesson 1: Embrace Aging

American Catholic nuns' "secret" to aging well is not what most of us embedded with antiaging cultural practices expect. The nuns do not avoid aging; they embrace it. While American cultural models measure "successful" aging by a yard stick designed to measure the maintenance of youth, the nuns aged well by embracing aging. The nuns teach us that feeling well, being healthy, and living longer lives involved embracing old age as a natural life stage. They did not expect older age to be an extension of younger adulthood; they embraced the age they were. They invested time and energy into learning how to be old gracefully. They embraced old age itself.

Lesson 2: Embrace Each Other

The nuns learned to embrace aging through social interaction. Together they valued communal living and serving others. If in older age a sister was not able to function independently, she could draw on a lifetime of experience living interdependently. This practice, relying on others and valuing interdependence, meant that the sisters did not interpret dependence as moral failure. Instead, when sisters grew older and had to depend on others for daily care, dependence seemed normal and good. Having served others all their lives, it was their turn to be embraced in service.

Lesson 3: Value Being, Not Doing

American cultural practices place value on productivity. Children are socialized from a young age to think about what they want to "do" when they grow up. As Jenny Odell writes about American culture, "In a world where our value is determined by our productivity, many of us find our every last minute captured, optimized, or appropriated as a financial resource" (2019, 1). For many people, the cultural value put on productivity can cause distress when bodily changes make it impossible to be productive. Many nuns faced anguish and self-judgment when they had to retire from a life of serving others and no longer felt that they were "doing good" in the world. Yet the cultural community of the convent met this challenge head-on by providing ongoing socialization to the sisters emphasizing that *being* good was just as important, if not more important, that *doing* good. The sisters continually reinforced the notion that they were valuable people even when they were not active. In this way the sisters taught each other how to value themselves at all stages of the life course, even in old age.

Lesson 4: Embrace All Persons

The nuns meaningfully engaged their peers even when they could not respond in kind. The sisters not only avoided elderspeak, the practice of speaking down to older adults, but engaged communicatively compromised older adults as respected peers, involving them in linguistically complex, grammatically rich interaction. This type of engagement can help individuals maintain their emotional and cognitive health. In addition, as we saw with Sister Helen's card games, women had ample opportunities to continue to engage in meaningful social activities instead of becoming socially isolated. The most important factor that made this type of engagement possible was the cultural value the nuns placed on all persons. Unlike their American lay peers, the nuns treated individuals as inherently valuable persons at all stages of life, not just when they were productive, independent adults. Because the nuns valued each other at all life stages, they embraced and engaged each other at all life stages. This had profound consequences for the well-being of those who grew older and for how younger nuns viewed their own future: they saw that if they developed dementia or other chronic conditions, they, too, would be respected, embraced, and engaged in their community.

Lesson 5: Language Is Powerful

The words the nuns spoke in prayer changed how they experienced both God and the world. This, in turn, shaped how they experienced their own bodies and pain. The words they spoke to each other about aging, healing, and death created a cultural context in which aging was experienced with grace and acceptance. What we say has the power to shape our experiences in the world. The words we speak each day matter; they represent our cultural values and also produce our cultural values. Listen to how you speak about aging. It has the power to reveal to you what might not yet be visible, and, like the nuns, together we have the power to create new cultural patterns through our language.

Lesson 6: Letting Go

Through habituated practices, the nuns trained themselves to respond to the inevitable losses that come with aging in the world with equanimity, acceptance, and relative peace. When the nuns were required to give up mobility or comfort as their bodies gave out in old age, they engaged in the same pattern, redirecting their attention from what they were giving up to focus on God's love. While the nuns' practices were rooted in Catholic theology, the empha-sis on letting go of attachments is paralleled in a number of traditions. For the nuns, a lifetime of practice in letting go of attachments helped them embrace the process of aging with equanimity and peace.

Lesson 7: The Body Is Social

While the cultural history that brought us the scientific tradition has illumi-nated a lot about the world we live in, human experience cannot be captured by numbers alone. Human life, how we experience the world, cannot be reduced to a data set. While Euro-American cultural traditions might imagine that the body is simply a material entity, the body is always embedded in a meaningful social world.[1] From the moment we are born, the body is imbued with mean-ing. Many scientific approaches may imagine the body as a solely material entity, for instance, measuring the things one puts in (kale, exercise, water, or wine) as connected to particular outputs (health, heart disease, and longevity). But our lives are not quite as simple as a set of material inputs and outputs. Our bodies are social. The nuns' stories demonstrate how profoundly the social world shapes the body. Their well-being is certainly impacted by material inputs such as what they eat, their relatively high level of education, and the fact that they never have to worry about having a roof over their head. But this book demonstrates that the story does not end there. How we age is connected to how we interact in the world. The social practices in which the nuns engaged shaped their health, their well-being, and their understanding of aging. How we age is interwoven with what aging means to each of us.

Appendix

• •

Transcription Conventions

?	a question mark indicates rising intonation
(1.0)	parentheses containing a number indicate a pause and the number of seconds
(.)	a period in parentheses indicates a micropause\, less than two-tenths of a second
.	a period indicates a falling intonation
__	word underlining indicates emphatic speech
::	a colon indicates a lengthening of the sound that precedes the colon. Two colons indicate an extended lengthening of the sound.
=	an equal sign indicates overlapping speech
( )	a pair of single parentheses with no text indicates a passage that was unclear in the recorded audio
(( ))	double parentheses indicate the author's description of affect/gesture and extended periods of laughter
(h)	h and variations in parentheses indicates laughter
boldface	boldface indicates a passage the author wishes to highlight for the reader
. . .	ellipses indicate lines were omitted from transcription

Acknowledgments

In the twelve years that I have been thinking and writing about how Catholic nuns support and care for each other, I have also been aware of enduring forms of support and care that have made my research possible.

First, I am grateful to Elinor Ochs, without whom I never would have thought to study Catholic convents. It was a blessing to have been your student at the University of California–Los Angeles, and I continue to feel deep joy and gratitude for your boundless support and encouragement. I am lucky to have spent many years under the insightful and affectionate care of one of our field's most creative and inspiring scholars. Thank you, Ellie, for inspiring me, challenging me, and supporting me throughout this process.

I am also grateful to Alessandro Duranti and Jason Throop, both of whom have influenced my intellectual orientation in the world. Sandro, thank you for teaching me how luxurious, inspiring, and fun it can be to soak up literature outside of our subfield. It was such a pleasure to watch you work. Jason, thank you for your concern, encouragement, and insights.

To Tanya Luhrmann, thank you for your generosity and inspiration. It has been such a delight to be invited into the intellectual world of cross-disciplinary scholarship you create and foster. I have had the most incredible conversations in your living room. Thank you for all you have done to push and support me.

Thank you also to my colleagues, peers, and friends who have made this process possible. I appreciate the encouragement, commiseration, laughter, and fantastic conversations. Thanks go especially to those who have been there from the very start—Katja Antoine, Keziah Conrad, Jenni Guzmán, Jessica Hardin, and Ellen Sharp.

Thank you, Jim Wilce, for introducing me to the field of anthropology. You kindled a fire that changed my life.

Thanks also to the generous souls who read drafts of this book: Anne Carpenter, Keziah Conrad, John Corwin, Jessica Hardin, Diana Insolio, Arlene Kahn, Irene Keenan, Tanya Luhrmann, Sylvia Lunt, David Magarian, Wayne Steele, Debbie Virga, and Carol Wong.

Thank you, Dana Herrera, for your unwavering support. Especially as I juggled editing the book with teaching and parenting in a pandemic, your support as department chair was extraordinary.

Thank you, Mom, for showing me by example that it is possible to be a good mother and to have a rigorous career. I apologize for all the times as a child that I pleaded with you to "'top 'tudying." I now know how painful it can be to tell your children that you have to work.

Thank you, Solomon and Luna Mae, for spending many of your formative months (both in utero and out) in the convent with me. You were each a big hit with the sisters. And thank you, David, for your undying support and for letting me take our first child away to a Catholic convent for the first months of his life. Thanks for coming with me and staying even after our neighbors called the cops on you when you took Solomon on a stroll. Your patience is inspiring. I could not have asked for a better partner.

The warmest of all thanks goes to everyone at the Franciscan Sisters of the Sacred Heart Convent. You took a big risk, letting a stranger into your homes and hearts. Thank you for trusting me with your lives and your stories. When I first conceived of this project, I never expected you to touch me so deeply. I am so lucky to have witnessed and experienced the love, kindness, warmth, and joy with which you live your lives.

I would also like to acknowledge the funding that facilitated this study: a National Science Foundation Dissertation Improvement Grant (ID #1026025), the UCLA Center for the Study of Women Jean Stone Dissertation Research Grant, and a fellowship from the National Endowment for the Humanities (HB-262298-19). Thank you for making this work possible.

Notes

Introduction

1 The United States, of course, is not the only society in which aging and decline are framed as problems in mainstream discourse. The devaluation of older adults and antiaging cultural practices more generally occur in various ways in a number of cultural communities around the world. For instance, in *The Coming of Age*, Simone de Beauvoir documents the social, political, and ideological forces in Europe that contribute to the cultural practices associated with devaluing older adults (1972, 37). Beauvoir writes, for instance, "society cares about the individual only in so far as he is profitable" (543). Nevertheless, as this book will demonstrate, the devaluation of older adults and the desire to avoid aging are cultural practices that are by no means universal. Anthropologists who study aging have shown that there is tremendous variation in how aging and the life course are understood and how older adults are valued and positioned. For instance, there are many communities in which older adults are respected, integrated in everyday activities, and aging and death are accepted (see, for example, Keith 1980; Keith et al. 1994; Lynch and Danely 2013; Sokolovsky 2009; Wilson 2000).

Chapter 1   Life in the Convent

1 Following IRB protocol, all of the sisters' names and the name of the convent have been changed in the interest of confidentiality.
2 I also spent time with Notre Dame Sisters in Los Angeles, in a Filles de Charité (Daughters of Charity) convent in Paris as well as with a contemplative Carmelite community in the Midwestern United States.
3 The postmaster once introduced herself to me as the only non-Catholic in town. She drove to the closest town, about fifteen minutes away, to attend a Baptist church.
4 Following IRB protocol, any identifying information has been removed from my transcripts in the interest of confidentiality.

Chapter 2   Being Is Harder Than Doing

1   I define the term *neoliberal* as pertaining to the ideologies and corresponding set of values and practices associated with free market capitalism. These values—which have imbued political, economic, and cultural practices across much of the globe—include ideals of freedom, independence, and autonomy.

2   As noted in the introduction, the United States is not the only society in which this paradigm dominates, however, as the ethnographic data were gathered in the United States, the book will focus on American cultural practices.

3   I use the terms *objective* and *subjective* here in loyalty to the literature I reference despite their troublesome assumptions. For a critique of this dichotomy, see Corwin and Erickson-Davis 2020.

4   Sixty-three nuns returned the survey. All participants answered the questions on psychological well-being. Only fifty-six of the sixty-three answered the questions on physical well-being.

5   The McGill Quality of Life Questionnaire asks psychological questions related to well-being such that the most desirable answers (no depression, for example), are rated 0. In Henry and colleagues' 2008 report, they transposed the descriptive statistics so that 10 was the most desirable score. Here I have reversed this transposition to match the way in which the questions were asked.

6   Some portions of this section were previously published in Corwin 2017.

7   Of course, the United States is not the only society that values productivity. As Max Weber traced in *The Protestant Ethic and the Spirit of Capitalism* in 1905, the values of productivity and the equation between work and morality emerged in Europe in the sixteenth century (Weber 2001 [1905]). In the United States, researchers have shown that Puritan values equating hard work, productivity, and morality continue to influence mainstream American cultural practices (See for example Amos, Zhang, and Read, 2019; Kang, 2009; Uhlmann, Poehlman, Tannenbaum and Bargh, 2011). For more reading on productivity and cultural practices in post-industrial United States, see Furnham et al., 1993 and Ochs and Kremer-Sadlik, 2013 and 2015.

Chapter 3   Talking to God

1   I have also written about this corpus of prayers in Corwin 2014.

Chapter 4   Care, Elderspeak, and Meaningful Engagement

1   A shorter version of this analysis appears Corwin 2018.

2   These data and analysis also appear in Corwin 2020.

Chapter 5   Changing God, Changing Bodies

1   A version of this chapter was previously published as Corwin 2012a.

Chapter 6   Spiritual Healing, Meaningful Decline, and Sister Death

1   For an examination of how these two traditions have come together in the United States, I recommend Swinton 2007 and Coblentz, forthcoming.

2   For a cross-cultural exploration of the intersection of faith and Christian salvation, see Hardin 2019.

Chapter 7   Kenosis

1   For an analysis of how to examine this presence, see Corwin and Erickson-Davis 2020.
2   Sister Marie is a composite portrait of three nuns. I have chosen to develop her in this way to protect the identity of the nuns who fit this portrait.

Conclusion

1   These themes are discussed in Heidegger 1962.

References

Abramson, Corey M. 2015. *The End Game: How Inequality Shapes Our Final Years*. Cambridge, MA: Harvard University Press.

Achenbaum, W. Andrew, and Vern L. Bengtson. 1994. "Re-engaging the Disengagement Theory of Aging: On the History and Assessment of Theory Development in Gerontology." *Gerontologist* 34: 756–763.

Agamben, Giorgio. 2013. *The Highest Poverty: Monastic Rules and Form-of-Life*. Translated by Adam Kotsko. Stanford, CA: Stanford University Press.

Amos, Clinton, Lixuan Zhang, and David Read. 2019. "Hardworking as a Heuristic for Moral Character: Why We Attribute Moral Values to Those Who Work Hard and Its Implications." *Journal of Business Ethics* 158 (4): 1047–1062.

Applewhite, Ashton. 2016. *This Chair Rocks: A Manifesto against Ageism*. New York: Celadon Books.

Asad, Talal. 1997. "Remarks on the Anthropology of the Body." In *Religion and the Body*, edited by Sarah Coakley, 42–52. Cambridge: Cambridge University Press.

Atkinson, J. Maxwell. 1984. *Our Masters' Voices: The Language and Body Language of Politics*. New York: Methuen.

Austin, J. L. 1962. *How to Do Things with Words*. Cambridge, MA: Harvard University Press.

Baltes, Paul B., and Margret M. Baltes. 1993a. "Psychological Perspectives on Successful Aging: The Model of Selective Optimization with Compensation." In *Successful Aging: Perspectives from the Behavioral Sciences*, edited by Paul B. Baltes and Margret M. Baltes, 1–34. New York: Cambridge University Press.

———, eds. 1993b. *Successful Aging: Perspectives from the Behavioral Sciences*. New York: Cambridge University Press.

Baquedano-Lopez, Patricia. 2000. "Narrating Community in Doctrina Classes." *Narrative Inquiry* 10 (2): 429–452.

Barsalou, Lawrence W., Aron K. Barbey, W. Kyle Simmons, and Ava Santos. 2005. "Embodiment in Religious Knowledge." *Journal of Cognition and Culture* 5 (1–2): 14–57.

Barss, M. Brooke. 2017. "Bearing Witness to Impermanence." MA Thesis, Upaya Zen Center.

Bastian, Brock, Jolanda Jetten, and Laura J. Ferris. 2014. "Pain as Social Glue: Shared Pain Increases Cooperation." *Psychological Science* 25 (11): 2079–2085.

Beauregard, Mario, and Vincent Paquette. 2006. "Neural Correlates of a Mystical Experience in Carmelite Nuns." *Neuroscience Letters* 405 (3): 186–190.

———. 2008. "EEG Activity in Carmelite Nuns during a Mystical Experience." *Neuroscience Letters* 444 (1): 1–4.

Beauvoir, Simone de. 1972. *The Coming of Age*. New York: Putnam.

Bell, Sandra, and Simon Coleman. 1999. *The Anthropology of Friendship*. London: Bloomsbury Academic.

Bendyna, Mary E., RSM, and Mary L. Gautier. 2009. *Recent Vocations to Religious Life: A Report for the National Religious Vocation Conference*. Washington, DC: Center for Applied Research in the Apostolate.

Benson, Bruce Ellis, and Norman Wirzba. 2005a. "Introduction." In *The Phenomenology of Prayer*, edited by Bruce Ellis Benson and Norman Wirzba, 1–10. New York: Fordham University Press.

———, eds. 2005b. *The Phenomenology of Prayer*. New York: Fordham University Press.

Berman, Elise. 2019. *Talking like Children: Language and the Production of Age in the Marshall Islands*. Oxford: Oxford University Press.

Berrelleza, Erick, Mary L. Gautier, and Mark M. Gray. 2014. *Population Trends among Religious Institutes of Women*. Washington, DC: Center for Applied Research in the Apostolate.

Bock, John, and Sara E. Johnson. 2004. "Play and Subsistence Ecology among the Okavango Delta." *Human Nature* 15 (1): 63–81.

Bourdieu, Pierre. 1990. *The Logic of Practice*. Translated by Richard Nice. Stanford, CA: Stanford University Press.

Briggs, Charles. 1993. "Personal Sentiments and Polyphonic Voices in Warao Women's Ritual Wailing: Music and Poetics in a Critical and Collective Discourse." *American Anthropologist* 95 (4): 929–995.

Bruder, Kurt A. 1998. "A Pragmatics for Human Relationship with the Divine: An Examination of the Monastic Blessing Sequence." *Journal of Pragmatics* 29: 463–491.

Buch, Elana D. 2013. "Senses of Care: Embodying Inequality and Sustaining Personhood in the Home Care of Older Adults in Chicago." *American Ethnologist* 40 (4): 637–650.

———. 2015. "Anthropology of Aging and Care." *Annual Review of Anthropology* 44: 277–293.

Buck, Joy. 2006. "Reweaving a Tapestry of Care: Religion, Nursing, and the Meaning of Hospice, 1945–1978." *Nursing History Review* 15 (1): 113–145.

Burt, Donald X. 1999. *Friendship and Society: An Introduction to Augustine's Practical Philosophy*. Grand Rapids, MI: William B. Eerdmans.

Butler, Robert N. 1975. *Why Survive? Being Old in America*. Oxford: Harper and Row.

Butler, Steven M., J. Wesson Ashford, and David A. Snowdon. 1996. "Age, Education, and Changes in the Mini-mental State Exam Scores of Older Women: Findings from the Nun Study." *Journal of the American Geriatrics Society* 44 (6), 675–681.

Butler, Steven M., and David A. Snowdon. 1996. "Trends in Mortality in Older Women: Findings from the Nun Study." *Journal of Gerontology: Social Sciences* 51B (4): S201–S208.

Calasanti, Toni. 2004. "Feminist Gerontology and Old Men." *Journals of Gerontology, Series B: Psychological Sciences and Social Sciences* 59 (6): S305–S314.

Capps, Lisa, and Elinor Ochs. 2002. "Cultivating Prayer." In *The Language of Turn and Sequence*, edited by Cecelia E. Ford, Barbara A. Fox, and Sandra A. Thompson, 39–55. Oxford: Oxford University Press.

Carlson, Charles R., Panayiota E. Bacaseta, and Dexter A. Simanton. 1988. "Controlled Evaluation of Devotional Meditation and Progressive Muscle Relaxation." *Journal of Psychology and Theology* 16 (4): 362–368.

Chapin, Bambi. 2014. *Childhood in a Sri Lankan Village: Shaping Hierarchy and Desire*. New Brunswick, NJ: Rutgers University Press.

Chittister, Joan. 2003. "The Struggle between Confusion and Expectation: The Legacy of Vatican II." In *Vatican II: Forty Personal Stories*, edited by Michael J. Daley and William Madges, 25–30. Mystic, CT: Twenty-Third.

———. 2010. *The Gift of Years: Growing Older Gracefully*. New York: BlueBridge.

Clifford, Catherine E. 2004. "Kenosis and the Path to Communion." *Jurist* 64: 21–34.

Coblentz, Jessica. Forthcoming. *Dust in the Blood: A Theology of Depression*. Collegeville, MN: Liturgical Academic Press.

Cohen, S. Robin, Balfour M. Mount, Eduardo Bruera, Marcel Provost, Jocelyn Rowe, and Kevin Tong. 1997. "Validity of the McGill Quality of Life Questionnaire in the Palliative Care Setting: A Multi-centre Canadian Study Demonstrating the Importance of the Existential Domain." *Palliative Medicine* 11 (3): 17–37.

Cohen, S. Robin, Balfour M. Mount, Michael G. Strobel, and France Bui. 1995. "The McGill Quality of Life Questionnaire: A Measure of Quality of Life Appropriate for People with Advanced Disease; A Preliminary Study of Validity and Acceptability." *Palliative Medicine* 9 (3): 207–219.

Cohen, Sheldon. 2004. "Social Relationships and Health." *American Psychologist* 59 (8): 676–684.

Cook, Joanna. 2010. *Meditation in Modern Buddhism*. New York: Cambridge University Press.

Coppens, Andrew D., Lucía Alcalá, Barbara Rogoff, and Rebeca Mejía-Arauz. 2018. "Children's Contributions in Family Work: Two Cultural Paradigms." In *Families, Intergenerationality, and Peer Group Relations*, edited by Samantha Punch, Robert Vanderbeck, and Tracey Skelton, 1–27. Singapore: Springer Singapore.

Corwin, Anna I. 2012a. "Changing God, Changing Bodies: The Impact of New Prayer Practices on Elderly Catholic Nuns' Embodied Experience." *Ethos* 40 (4): 390–410.

———. 2012b. "Let Him Hold You: Spiritual and Social Support in a Catholic Convent Infirmary." *Anthropology of Aging Quarterly* 33 (4): 120–130.

———. 2014. "Lord, Hear Our Prayer: Prayer, Social Support, and Well-Being in a Catholic Convent." *Journal of Linguistic Anthropology* 24 (2): 174–192.

———. 2017. "Growing Old with God: An Alternative Vision of Aging Well." In *Successful Aging as a Contemporary Obsession*, edited by Sarah Lamb, 98–111. New Brunswick, NJ: Rutgers University Press.

———. 2018. "Overcoming Elderspeak: A Qualitative Study of Three Alternatives." *Gerontologist* 58 (4): 724–729.

———. 2020. "Care in Interaction: Aging, Personhood, and Meaningful Decline." *Medical Anthropology: Cross-Cultural Studies in Health and Illness* 39 (7): 638–652.

Corwin, Anna I., and Cordelia Erickson-Davis. 2020. "Experiencing Presence: An Interactive Model of the Divine." *HAU: Journal of Ethnographic Theory* 10 (1): 166–182.

Courtin, Emilie, and Martin Knapp. 2015. "Social Isolation, Loneliness and Health in Old Age: A Scoping Review." *Health and Social Care in the Community* 25 (3): 799–812.

Cronin, Kevin M. 1992. *Kenosis: Emptying Self and the Path of Christian Service.* New York: Continuum.

Csordas, Thomas J. 1993. "Somatic Modes of Attention." *Cultural Anthropology* 8 (2): 135–156.

———. 1994. *The Sacred Self: A Cultural Phenomenology of Charismatic Healing.* Berkeley: University of California Press.

———. 2008. "Intersubjectivity and Intercorporeality." *Subjectivity* 22 (1): 110–121.

Cumming, Elaine, and William Henry. 1961. *Growing Old: The Process of Disengagement.* New York: Basic Books.

Cunningham, Jacqueline, and Kristine N. Williams. 2007. "A Case Study of Resistiveness to Care and Elderspeak." *Research and Theory for Nursing Practice* 21 (12): 45–56.

Danner, Deborah D., David A. Snowdon, and Wallace V. Friesen. 2001. "Positive Emotions in Early Life and Longevity: Findings from the Nun Study." *Journal of Personality and Social Psychology* 80 (5): 804–813.

Dein, Simon. 2002. "The Power of Words: Healing Narratives among Lubavitcher Hasidim." *Medical Anthropology Quarterly* 16 (2): 41–63.

Diener, Ed, and Micaela Y. Chan. 2011. "Happy People Live Longer: Subjective Well-Being Contributes to Health and Longevity." *Applied Psychology: Health and Well-Being* 3 (1): 1–43.

Dillaway, Heather E., and Mary Byrnes. 2009. "Reconsidering Successful Aging: A Call for Renewed and Expanded Academic Critiques and Conceptualizations." *Journal of Applied Gerontology* 28 (6): 702–722.

Donohoe, Martin. 2012. *Public Health and Social Justice.* New York: John Wiley and Sons.

Dreyfus, Georges B. J. 2003. *The Sound of Two Hands Clapping: The Education of a Tibetan Buddhist Monk.* Berkeley: University of California Press.

Durkheim, Émile. 1912. *Les formes élémentaires de la vie religieuse.* Paris: Alcan.

Edwards, Helen, and Patricia Noller. 1993. "Perceptions of Overaccommodation Used by Nurses in Communication with the Elderly." *Journal of Language and Social Psychology* 12 (3): 207–223.

Evans, Gary W., and Elyse Kantrowitz. 2002. "Socioeconomic Status and Health: The Potential Role of Environmental Risk Exposure." *Annual Review of Public Health* 23 (1): 303–331.

Fabbre, Vanessa D. 2014. "Gender Transitions in Later Life: A Queer Perspective on Successful Aging." *Gerontologist* 55 (1): 144–153.

Ferguson, Charles A. 1985. "The Study of Religious Discourse." In *Languages and Linguistics: The Interdependence of Theory, Data, and Application*, edited by Deborah Tannon and James Atalis, 205–213. Washington, DC: Georgetown University Press.

Fisher, Linda. 2015. "The Illness Experience." In *Feminist Phenomenology and Medicine*, edited by Kristin J. Zeiler and Lisa Folkmarson Käll, 27–46. Albany: State University of New York Press.

Foucault, Michel. 1988. "Technologies of the Self." In *Technologies of the Self: A Seminar with Michel Foucault*, edited by Luther H. Martin, Huck Gutman, and Patrick H. Hutton, 16–49. Amherst: University of Massachusetts Press.

Furnham, Adrian, Michael Bond, Patrick Heaven, Denis Hilton, Thalma Lobel, John Masters, Monica Payne, R. Rajamanikam, Barrie Stacey, and H. Van Daalen. 1993. "A Comparison of Protestant Work Ethic Beliefs in Thirteen Nations." *Journal of Social Psychology* 133 (2): 185–197.

Garrett, Paul B., and Patricia Baquedano-Lopez. 2002. "Language Socialization: Reproduction and Continuity, Transformation and Change." *Annual Review of Anthropology* 31: 339–361.

Gautier, Mary L., and Carolyne Saunders. 2013. *New Sisters and Brothers Professing Perpetual Vows in Religious Life*. Washington, DC: Center for Applied Research in the Apostolate.

Gee, Gilbert C., and Devon C. Payne-Sturges. 2004. "Environmental Health Disparities: A Framework Integrating Psychosocial and Environmental Concepts." *Environmental Health Perspectives* 112 (17): 1645–1653.

Gingrich, Andre, Elinor Ochs, and Alan Swedlund. 2002. "Repertoires of Timekeeping in Anthropology." *Current Anthropology* 43 (S4): S3–S4.

Globe Newswire. "Anti-Aging Products Industry Projected to be Worth $83.2 Billion by 2027: Key Trends, Opportunities and Players." July 24, 2020. https://www.globenewswire.com/news-release/2020/07/24/2067180/0/en/Anti-Aging-Products-Industry-Projected-to-be-Worth-83-2-Billion-by-2027-Key-Trends-Opportunities-and-Players.html#:~:text=The%20Anti%2DAging%20Products%20market, share%20in%20the%20global%20market.&text=Among%20the%20other%20noteworthy%20geographic,over%20the%202020%2D2027%20period

Goffman, Erving. 1961. *Asylums: Essays on the Social Situation of Mental Patients and Other Inmates*. New York: Anchor Books.

Golden, Jeannette, Ronán M. Conroy, Irene Bruce, Aisling Denihan, Elaine Greene, Michael Kirby, and Brian A. Lawlor. 2009. "Loneliness, Social Support Networks, Mood and Wellbeing in Community-Dwelling Elderly." *International Journal of Geriatric Psychiatry* 24 (7): 694–700.

Golden, Jeannette, Ronán M. Conroy, and Brian A. Lawlor. 2009. "Social Support Network Structure in Older People: Underlying Dimensions and Association with Psychological and Physical Health." *Psychology, Health and Medicine* 14 (3): 280–290.

Good, Mary-Jo DelVecchio, Paul Brodwin, Byron Good, and Arthur Kleinman. 1994. *Pain as Human Experience*. Berkeley: University of California Press.

Gottlieb, Benjamin H. 1985. "Social Networks and Social Support: An Overview of Research, Practice, and Policy Implications." *Health Education and Behavior* 12 (5): 5–22.

Gould, Odette N., Cybil Saum, and Jennifer Belter. 2002. "Recall and Subjective Reactions to Speaking Styles: Does Age Matter?" *Experimental Aging Research* 28 (2): 199–213.

Grainger, Karen. 1993. "'That's a Lovely Bath Dear': Reality Construction in the Discourse of Elderly Care." *Journal of Aging Studies* 7 (3): 247–262.

Greenblatt, Stephen. 2011. *The Swerve: How the World Became Modern*. New York: W. W. Norton.

Grice, Paul. 1989. *Studies in the Way of Words*. Cambridge, MA: Harvard University Press.

Gross, Jane. 2011. *A Bittersweet Season: Caring for Our Aging Parents—and Ourselves.* New York: Vintage Books.

Hanks, William. 1996. *Language and Communicative Practice.* Boulder, CO: Westview.

Hardin, Jessica. 2019. *Faith and the Pursuit of Health: Cardiometabolic Disorders in Samoa.* New Brunswick, NJ: Rutgers University Press.

Harding, Susan Friend. 2000. *The Book of Jerry Falwell: Fundamentalist Language and Politics.* Princeton, NJ: Princeton University Press.

Hauerwas, Stanley. 2004. *Naming the Silences: God, Medicine, and the Problem of Suffering.* New York: T&T Clark.

Havighurst, Robert J. 1961. "Successful Aging." *Gerontologist* 1 (1): 8–13.

Hawkley, Louise C., John T. Cacioppo. 2010. "Loneliness Matters: A Theoretical and Empirical Review of Consequences and Mechanisms." *Annals of Behavioral Medicine* 40 (2): 218–227.

Heidegger, Martin. 1962. *Being and Time.* Translated by John Macquarrie and Edward Robinson. New York: Harper and Row.

Heil, Daniela. 2010. "Embodied Selves and Social Selves: Aboriginal Well-Being in Rural New South Wales, Australia." In *Pursuits of Happiness: Well-Being in Anthropological Perspective*, edited by Gordon Mathews and Carolina Izquierdo, 88–108. New York: Berghahn Books.

Helmstadter, Carol, and Judith Godden. 2016. *Nursing before Nightingale, 1815–1899.* New York: Routledge.

Henry, Melissa, Lina Nuoxin Huang, Mira Klode Ferland, Julie Mitchell, and S. Robin Cohen. 2008. "Continued Study of the Psychometric Properties of the McGill Quality of Life Questionnaire." *Palliative Medicine* 22: 718–723.

Hill, Patrick L., Grant W. Edmonds, and Sarah E. Hampson. 2017. "A Purposeful Lifestyle Is a Healthful Lifestyle: Linking Sense of Purpose to Self-Rated Health through Multiple Health Behaviors." *Journal of Health Psychology* 24 (10): 1392–1400.

Hirschkind, Charles. 2001. "The Ethics of Listening: Cassette-Sermon Audition in Contemporary Egypt." *American Ethnologist* 28 (3): 623–649.

Hollan, Douglas. 2010. "Selfscapes of Well-Being in a Rural Indonesian Village." In *Pursuits of Happiness: Well-Being in Anthropological Perspective*, edited by Gordon Mathews and Carolina Izquierdo, 21–27. New York: Berghahn Books.

Ikeuchi, Suma. 2017. "Accompanied Self: Debating Pentecostal Individual and Japanese Relational Selves in Transnational Japan." *Ethos* 45 (1): 3–23.

Izquierdo, Carolina. 2010. "Well-Being among the Matsigenka of the Peruvian Amazon: Health, Missions, Oil, and 'Progress.'" In *Pursuits of Happiness: Well-Being in Anthropological Perspective*, edited by Gordon Mathews and Carolina Izquierdo, 67–87. New York: Berghahn Books.

Jacoby, Sally, and Patrick Gonzales. 1991. "The Constitution of Expert-Novice in Scientific Discourse." *Issues in Applied Linguistics* 2 (2): 149–181.

Jakobson, Roman. 1987. "Poetry of Grammar and Grammar of Poetry." In *Language in Literature*, edited by Krysyna Pomorska and Stephen Rudy, 121–144. Cambridge, MA: Belknap.

James, William. 1982. *The Varieties of Religious Experience.* New York: Penguin.

Julian of Norwich. 1998. *Revelations of Divine Love.* Translated by Elizabeth Spearing. London: Penguin.

Kalb, Dan. 2018. "Why I Will Not Make It as a 'Moral Anthropologist.'" In *Moral Anthropology: A Critique*, edited by Bruce Kapferer and Marina Gold, 65–76. New York: Berghahn Books.

Kang, Ning. 2009. "Puritanism and Its Impact upon American Values." *Review of European Studies* 1: 148.

Kapferer, Bruce, and Marina Gold. 2018a. "Introduction: Reconceptualizing the Discipline." In *Moral Anthropology: A Critique*, edited by Bruce Kapferer and Marina Gold, 1–24. New York: Berghahn Books.

———, eds. 2018b. *Moral Anthropology: A Critique*. New York: Berghahn Books.

Kaplan, George A., Gavin Turrell, John W. Lynch, Susan A. Everson, Eeva-Liisa Helkala, and Jukka T. Salonen. 2001. "Childhood Socioeconomic Position and Cognitive Function in Adulthood." *International Journal of Epidemiology* 30 (2): 256–263.

Keane, Webb. 1997. "Religious Language." *Annual Review of Anthropology* 26: 47–71.

Keith, Jennie. 1980. "'The Best Is Yet To Be': Toward an Anthropology of Age." *Annual Review of Anthropology* 9 (1): 339–364.

Keith, Jennie, Christine L. Fry, Anthony P. Glascock, Charlotte Ikels, Jeanette Dickerson-Putman, Henry C. Harpending, and Patricia Draper. 1994. *The Aging Experience: Diversity and Commonality across Cultures*. London. Sage Publications.

Kemper, Susan, and Tamara Harden. 1999. "Experimentally Disentangling What's Beneficial about Elderspeak from What's Not." *Psychology and Aging* 14 (4): 656–670.

Kittay, Eva Feder. 2010. "At the Margins of Moral Personhood." *Ethics* 116 (1): 100–131.

Kleinman, Arthur, Paul E. Brodwin, Mary-Jo DelVecchio Good, and Byron J. Good. 1994. "Pain as Human Experience: An Introduction." In *Pain as Human Experience: An Anthropological Perspective*, 1–28. Berkeley: University of California Press.

Koenig, Harold G. 1999. *The Healing Power of Faith: Science Explores Medicine's Last Great Frontier*. New York: Simon and Schuster.

———. 2003. *Chronic Pain: Biomedical and Spiritual Approaches*. Binghamton, NY: Hawthorne Pastoral Press.

Koenig, Harold G., Harold Jay Cohen, Linda K. George, Judith C. Hays, David B. Larson, and Dan G. Blazer. 1997. "Attendance at Religious Services, Interleukin-6, and Other Biological Parameters of Immune Function in Older Adults." *International Journal of Psychiatry in Medicine* 27 (3): 233–250.

Lamb, Sarah. 1997. "The Making and Unmaking of Persons: Notes on Aging and Gender in North India." *Ethos* 25 (3): 279–302.

———. 2000. *White Saris and Sweet Mangoes: Aging, Gender, and Body in North India*. Berkeley: University of California Press.

———. 2009. *Aging and the Indian Diaspora: Cosmopolitan Families in India and Abroad*. Bloomington: Indiana University Press.

———. 2014. "Permanent Personhood or Meaningful Decline? Toward a Critical Anthropology of Successful Aging." *Journal of Aging Studies* 29: 41–52.

Lamb, Sarah, Jessica Robbins-Ruszkowski, and Anna I. Corwin. 2017. "Introduction: Successful Aging as a 21st Century Obsession." In *Successful Aging as a Contemporary Obsession*, edited by Sarah Lamb, 1–26. New Brunswick, NJ: Rutgers University Press.

Lancy, David F. 2015. *The Anthropology of Childhood: Cherubs, Chattel, Changelings*. 2nd ed. Cambridge: Cambridge University Press.

Lester, Rebecca J. 2005. *Jesus in Our Wombs: Embodying Modernity in a Mexican Convent.* Berkeley: University of California Press.

Levy, Robert I., and Douglas Hollan. 1998. "Person-Centered Interviewing and Observation." In *Handbook of Methods in Cultural Anthropology,* edited by H. Russell Bernard, 333–364. Walnut Creek, CA: Altamira.

Liang, Jiayin, and Baozhen Luo. 2012. "Toward a Discourse Shift in Social Gerontology: From Successful Aging to Harmonious Aging." *Journal of Aging Studies* 26 (3): 327–334.

Lichtmann, Maria R. 1991. "'I Desyrede a Bodylye Syght': Julian of Norwich and the Body." *Mystics Quarterly* 17 (1): 12–19.

Lim, Chaeyoon, and Robert Putman. 2010. "Religion, Social Networks, and Life Satisfaction." *American Sociological Review* 75 (6): 914–933.

Lucy, John A. 1992. *Language Diversity and Thought.* Cambridge: Cambridge University Press.

———. 1997. "Linguistic Relativity." *Annual Review of Anthropology* 26 (1): 291–312.

Luhrmann, Tanya M. 2004. "Metakinesis: How God Becomes Intimate in Contemporary US Christianity." American Anthropologist 106 (3): 518–528.

———. 2005. "The Art of Hearing God: Absorption, Dissociation, and Contemporary American Spirituality." *Spiritus* 5 (2): 133–157.

———. 2012. *When God Talks Back: Understanding the American Evangelical Relationship with God.* New York: Random House.

Luhrmann, Tanya M., Howard Nusbaum, and Ronald Thisted. 2010. "The Absorption Hypothesis: Learning to Hear God in Evangelical Christianity." *American Anthropologist* 112 (1): 66–79.

Lynch, Caitrin, and Jason Danely, eds. 2013. *Transitions and Transformations: Cultural Perspectives on Aging and the Life Course.* New York. Berghahn Books.

Manderson, Lenore, and Carolyn Smith-Morris. 2010. *Chronic Conditions, Fluid States: Chronicity and the Anthropology of Illness.* New Brunswick, NJ: Rutgers University Press.

Margai, Florence. 2013. *Environmental Health Hazards and Social Justice: Geographical Perspectives.* New York: Routledge.

Marmot, Michael G., Manolis Kogevinas, and Mary Alan Elston. 1987. "Social/Economic Status and Disease." *Annual Review of Public Health* 8 (1): 111–135.

Martin, Emily. 1994. *Flexible Bodies: Tracking Immunity in American Culture—from the Days of Polio to the Age of AIDS.* Boston: Beacon.

Mathews, Gordon, and Carolina Izquierdo. 2010a. "Introduction: Anthropology, Happiness, and Well-Being." In *Pursuits of Happiness: Well-Being in Anthropological Perspective,* edited by Gordon Mathews and Carolina Izquierdo, 1–22. New York: Berghahn Books.

———, eds. 2010b. *Pursuits of Happiness: Well-Being in Anthropological Perspective.* New York: Berghahn Books.

Maton, Kenneth I. 1989. "The Stress-Buffering Role of Spiritual Support: Cross-Sectional and Prospective Investigation." *Journal for the Scientific Study of Religion* 28 (3): 310–323.

Mayne, Stephanie L., Margaret T. Hicken, Sharon Stein Merkin, Teresa E. Seeman, Kiarri N. Kershaw, D. Phuong Do, Anjum Hajat, and Ana V. Diez Roux. 2019. "Neighbourhood Racial/Ethnic Residential Segregation and Cardiometabolic Risk: The Multiethnic Study of Atherosclerosis." *Journal of Epidemiology and Community Health* 73 (1): 26–33.

McGrath, Patricia A. 1990. *Pain in Children: Nature, Assessment, and Treatment.* New York: Guilford.

McNamara, Patrick. 2009. *The Neuroscience of Religious Experience.* New York: Cambridge University Press.

McNamara, Patrick, and P. Monroe Butler. 2014. "The Neuropsychology of Religious Experience." In *Handbook of the Psychology of Religion and Spirituality*, edited by Raymond F. Paloutzian and Crystal L. Park, 215–233. New York: Guilford.

Mensch, James. 2005. "Prayer as Kenosis." In *The Phenomenology of Prayer*, edited by Bruce Ellis Benson and Norman Wirzba, 63–74. New York: Fordham University Press.

Merton, Thomas. 1961. *New Seeds of Contemplation.* New York: New Directions.

Millett, Bella, trans. 2009. *Ancrene Wisse / Guide for Anchoresses: A Translation.* Exeter, UK: University of Exeter Press.

Morinis, Alan. 1985. "The Ritual Experience." *Ethos* 13 (2): 150–174.

Morris, David B. 1991. *The Culture of Pain.* Berkeley: University of California Press.

Mortimer, James A., David A. Snowdon, and William R. Markesbery. 2003. "Head Circumference, Education and Risk of Dementia: Findings from the Nun Study." *Journal of Clinical and Experimental Neuropsychology* 25 (5): 671–679.

National Council on Aging. "Chronic Disease Management." Accessed February 9, 2021. https://www.ncoa.org/healthy-aging/chronic-disease/

Newberg, Andrew, with Mark Robert Waldman. 2006. *Why We Believe What We Believe: Uncovering Our Biological Need for Meaning, Spirituality, and Truth.* New York: Free Press.

Newberg, Andrew B., Nancy Wintering, Mark R. Waldman, Daniel Amen, Dharma S. Khalsa, and Abass Alavi. 2010a. "Cerebral Blood Flow Differences between Long-Term Meditators and Non-Meditators." *Consciousness and Cognition* 19 (4): 899–905.

———. 2010b. "The Measurement of Regional Cerebral Blood Flow during Glossolalia: A Preliminary SPECT Study." *Psychiatry Research* 148 (1): 67–71.

Norris, Rebecca Sachs. 2009. "The Paradox of Healing Pain." *Religion* 39 (1): 22–33.

Nussbaum, Jon F., Mary Lee Hummert, Angie Williams, and Jake Harwood. 1996. "Communication and Older Adults." *Annals of the International Communication Association* 19 (1): 1–48.

Ochs, Elinor. 1979. "Transcription as Theory." In *Developmental Pragmatics*, edited by Elinor Ochs and Bambi Schieffelin, 43–72. New York: Academic Press.

———. 2012. "Experiencing Language." *Anthropological Theory* 12 (2): 142–160.

Ochs, Elinor, and Lisa Capps. 2001. *Living Narrative: Creating Lives in Everyday Storytelling.* Cambridge, MA: Harvard University Press.

Ochs, Elinor, and Carolina Izquierdo. 2009. "Responsibility in Childhood: Three Developmental Trajectories." *Ethos* 37 (4): 391–413.

Ochs, Elinor, and Tamar Kremer-Sadlik. 2013. *Fast-forward Family: Home, Work, and Relationships in Middle-Class America.* Berkeley: University of California Press.

———. 2015. "How Postindustrial Families Talk." *Annual Review of Anthropology* 44: 87–103.

Ochs, Elinor, and Bambi Schieffelin. 1984. "Language Acquisition and Socialization: Three Developmental Stories and Their Implications." In *Culture Theory Essays on Mind, Self, and Emotion*, edited by Richard A. Shweder and Robert Alan LeVine, 276–320. Cambridge: Cambridge University Press.

Odell, Jenny. 2019. *How to Do Nothing: Resisting the Attention Economy.* Brooklyn, NY: Melville House.

O'Malley, John W. 2008. *What Happened at Vatican II*. Cambridge, MA: Belknap.

Ong, Anthony D., Burt N. Uchino, and Elaine Wethington. 2016. "Loneliness and Health in Older Adults: A Mini-review and Synthesis." *Gerontology* 62 (4): 443–449.

Orsi, Robert A. 2005. *Between Heaven and Earth: The Religious Worlds People Make and the Scholars Who Study Them*. Princeton, NJ: Princeton University Press.

Paradise, Ruth, and Barbara Rogoff. 2009. "Side by Side: Learning by Observing and Pitching in." *Ethos* 37 (1): 102–138.

Perkins, Judith. 2002. *The Suffering Self: Pain and Narrative Representation in the Early Christian Era*. London: Routledge.

Pevey, Carolyn F., Thomas J. Jones, and Annice Yarber. 2008. "How Religion Comforts the Dying: A Qualitative Inquiry." *Omega* 58 (1): 41–59.

Pincikowski, Scott E. 2013. *Bodies of Pain*. London: Routledge.

Prejean, Helen. 2019. "Sister Helen Prejean on Witnessing Executions: 'I Couldn't Let Them Die Alone.'" *Fresh Air*, August 12, 2019. https://www.npr.org/templates /transcript/transcript.php?storyId=750470040.

Prigerson, Holly Gwen. 1992. "Socialization to Dying: Social Determinants of Death Acknowledgement and Treatment among Terminally Ill Geriatric Patients." *Journal of Health and Social Behavior* 33 (4): 378–395.

Pryce, Paula. 2017. *The Monk's Cell*. Oxford: Oxford University Press.

Ralph, Margaret Nutting. 2003. *And God Said What? An Introduction to Biblical Literary Forms*. Mahwah, NJ: Paulist Press.

Riley, Kathryn P., David A. Snowdon, and William R. Markesbery. 2002. "Alzheimer's Neurofibrillary Pathology and the Spectrum of Cognitive Function: Findings from the Nun Study." *Annals of Neurology* 51 (5): 567–577.

Robbins, Joel. 2007. "Continuity, Thinking and the Problem of Christian Culture: Belief, Time, and the Anthropology of Christianity." *Current Anthropology* 48 (1): 5–38.

———. 2013. "Beyond the Suffering Subject: Toward an Anthropology of the Good." *Journal of the Royal Anthropological Institute* 19 (3): 447–462.

Rogoff, Barbara. 2003. *The Cultural Nature of Human Development*. Oxford: Oxford University Press.

Rowe, John, and Robert Kahn. 1997. "Successful Aging." *Gerontologist* 37 (4): 433–440.

———. 1998. *Successful Aging*. New York: Dell.

Ruether, Rosemary Radford. 1991. "The Place of Women in the Church." In *Modern Catholicism: Vatican II and After*, edited by Adrian Hastings, 260–266. New York: Oxford University Press.

Rupp, Joyce. 2007. *Prayer*. Maryknoll, NY: Orbis.

Ryan, Ellen Bouchard, Mary Lee Hummert, and Linda H. Boich. 1995. "Communication Predicaments of Aging: Patronizing Behavior toward Older Adults." *Journal of Language and Social Psychology* 14 (1–2): 144–166.

Ryan, Ellen Bouchard, Maryanne Maclean, and J. B. Orange. 1994. "Inappropriate Accommodation in Communication to Elders: Inferences about Nonverbal Correlates." *International Journal of Aging and Human Development* 39 (4): 273–291.

Saint Augustine. 1954. *The Confessions of St. Augustine*. London: Burns and Oates.

Saint Benedict. 1984. *The Rule of Saint Benedict*. London: Darton, Longman and Todd.

Saint Gregory the Great. 2010. *Dialogues*. Vol. 39, *The Fathers of the Church*. Catholic University of America Press.

Salsman, John M., Tamara L. Brown, Emily H. Brechting, and Charles R. Carlson. 2005. "The Link between Religion and Spirituality and Psychological Adjustment: The Mediating Role of Optimism and Social Support." *Personality and Social Psychology Bulletin* 31 (4): 522–533.

Salthouse, Timothy A. 1999. "Theories of Cognition." In *Handbook of Theories of Aging*, edited by Vern Bengston and Richard Stetteron, 196–208. New York: Springer.

Savage, Sharon A., Olivier Piguet, and John R. Hodges. 2015. "Cognitive Intervention in Semantic Dementia: Maintaining Words over Time." *Alzheimer Disease and Associated Disorders* 29 (1): 55–62.

Schieffelin, Bambi B., and Elinor Ochs. 1986. "Language Socialization." *Annual Review of Anthropology* 15 (1): 163–191.

Seeman, Teresa E. 1996. "Social Ties and Health: The Benefits of Social Integration." *Annals of Epidemiology* 6 (5): 442–451.

Seligman, Rebecca. 2010. "The Unmaking and Making of Self: Embodied Suffering and Mind–Body Healing in Brazilian Candomble." *Ethos* 38 (3): 297–320.

Shilling, Chris, and Philip A. Mellor. 2010. "Saved from Pain or Saved through Pain? Modernity, Instrumentalization and the Religious Use of Pain as a Body Technique." *European Journal of Social Theory* 13 (4): 521–537.

Shippee, Tetyana Pylypiv. 2009. "'But I Am Not Moving': Residents' Perspectives on Transitions within a Continuing Care Retirement Community." *Gerontologist* 49 (3): 418–427.

Shoaps, Robin. 2002. "'Pray Earnestly': The Textual Construction of Personal Involvement in Pentecostal Prayer and Song." *Journal of Linguistic Anthropology* 12 (1): 34–71.

Simon, Gregory M. 2009. "The Soul Freed of Cares? Islamic Prayer, Subjectivity, and the Contradictions of Moral Selfhood in Minangkabau, Indonesia." *American Ethnologist* 36 (2): 258–275.

Snowdon, David. 2001. *Aging with Grace: What the Nun Study Teaches Us about Leading Longer, Healthier, and More Meaningful Lives*. New York: Bantam Books.

Snowdon, David A., Susan Kemper, James Mortimer, Lydia Greiner, David R. Wekstein, and William R. Mardesbery. 1996. "Linguistic Ability in Early Life and Cognitive Function and Alzheimer's Disease in Late Life: Findings from the Nun Study." *Journal of the American Medical Association* 275 (7): 528–533.

Snowdon, David A., Sharon K. Ostwald, and Robert L. Kane. 1989. "Education, Survival, and Independence in Elderly Catholic Sisters, 1936–1988." *American Journal of Epidemiology* 130 (5): 999–1012.

Snowdon, David A., Christine L. Tully, Charles D. Smith, Kathryn Perez Riley, and William R. Markesbery. 2000. "Serum Folate and the Severity of Atrophy of the Neocortex in Alzheimer Disease: Findings from the Nun Study." *American Journal of Clinical Nutrition* 71 (4): 993–998.

Sokolovsky, Jay, ed. 2009. *The Cultural Context of Aging: Worldwide Perspectives*. Santa Barbara, CA. Praeger Publishers/Greenwood Publishing Group.

Soine, Aeleah. 2009. "From Nursing Sisters to a Sisterhood of Nurses: German Nurses and Transnational Professionalization, 1836–1918." PhD diss., University of Minnesota.

Starrett, Gregory. 1995. "The Hexis of Interpretation: Islam and the Body in the Egyptian Popular School." *American Ethnologist* 22 (4): 953–969.

Strawbridge, William, Richard D. Cohen, Sarah J. Shema, and George A. Kaplan. 1997. "Frequent Attendance at Religious Services and Mortality over 28 Years." *American Journal of Public Health* 87 (6): 957–961.

Stetler, Emily M. 2012. "Poured Out like an Offering: Toward an Anthropology of Kenosis." PhD diss., University of Notre Dame.

Swinton, John. 2013. *Raging with Compassion: Pastoral Responses to the Problem of Evil.* Grand Rapids, MI: William B. Eerdmans.

Tanquerey, Adolphe. 1930. *The Spiritual Life: A Treatise on Ascetical and Mystical Theology.* Tournai, Belgium: Society of St. John the Evangelist.

Thoits, Peggy A. 1995. "Stress, Coping, and Social Support Processes: Where Are We? What Next?" *Journal of Health and Social Behavior* 35: 53–79.

Throop, C. Jason. 2008. "From Pain to Virtue: Dysphoric Sensations and Moral Sensibilities in Yap (Waqab), Federated States of Micronesia." *Journal of Transcultural Psychiatry* 45 (2): 253–286.

———. 2010. *Suffering and Sentiment: Exploring the Vicissitudes of Experience and Pain in Yap.* Berkeley: University of California Press.

Time. 2001. Cover. *Time*, May 14, 2001. http://content.time.com/time/magazine/0,9263,7601010514,00.html

Turner, Bryan S. 1997. "The Body in Western Society: Social Theory and Its Perspectives." In *Religion and the Body*, edited by Sarah Coakley, 15–41. Cambridge: Cambridge University Press.

Uhlmann, Eric Luis, T. Andrew Poehlman, David Tannenbaum, and John A. Bargh. 2011. "Implicit Puritanism in American Moral Cognition." *Journal of Experimental Social Psychology* 47 (2): 312–320.

University of East Anglia. 2019. "Eating Blueberries Every Day Improves Heart Health." MedicalXpress, May 30, 2019. https://medicalxpress.com/news/2019-05-blueberries-day-heart-health.html.

Urban, Gregory. 1988. "Ritual Wailing in Amerindian Brazil." *American Anthropologist* 90 (2): 385–400.

Van Riessen, Renée D. N. 2007. *Man as a Place of God: Levinas' Hermeneutics of Kenosis.* Dordrecht, Netherlands: Springer.

Vatican Council. 1965. *Decree on the Adaptation and Renewal of Religious Life: Perfectae Caritatis.* October 28, 1965. N.p.: St. Paul Editions. http://www.vatican.va/archive/hist_councils/ii_vatican_council/documents/vat-ii_decree_19651028_perfectae-caritatis_en.html. Accessed Feb. 5, 2021.

Vos, Casparus Johannes Adam. 2005. *Theopoetry of the Psalms.* Pretoria, South Africa: Protea.

Weaver, Mary Jo. 1999. "American Catholics in the Twentieth Century." In *Perspectives on American Religion and Culture*, edited by Peter W. Williams, 154–167. Malden, MA: Blackwell.

Weber, Max. 2001 [1905]. *The Protestant Ethic and the Spirit of Capitalism.* Translated by Stephen Kalberg. Chicago: Fitzroy Dearborn Publishers.

Weisner, Thomas. 1998. "Human Development, Child Well-Being, and the Cultural Project of Development." *New Directions for Child and Adolescent Development* 80: 69–85.

———. 2002. "Ecocultural Understanding of Children's Developmental Pathways." *Human Development* 45: 275–281.

Westphal, Merold. 2005. "Prayer as the Posture of the Decentered Self." In *The Phenomenology of Prayer*, edited by Bruce Ellis Benson and Norman Wirzba, 13–31. New York: Fordham University Press.

Wilson, Gail. 2000. *Understanding Old Age: Critical and Global Perspectives*. London: Sage Publications.

Whiting, John W. M., Richard Kluckhohn, and Albert Anthony. 1958. "The Function of Male Initiation Ceremonies at Puberty." In *Readings in Social Psychology*, edited by Eleanor E. Macoby, Theodore M. Newcomb, and Eugene L. Hartley, 359–370. New York: Henry R. Holt.

Whorf, Benjamin Lee. 1956. "Language, Thought, and Reality: Selected Writings." Edited by John B. Carroll. Cambridge, MA: MIT Press.

———. 1997. "The Relation of Habitual Thought and Behavior to Language." In *Sociolinguistics: A Reader*, edited by Nikolas Coupland and Adam Jaworski, 443–463. London: Palgrave.

Williams, Kristine, Susan Kemper, and Mary Lee Hummert. 2003. "Improving Nursing Home Communication: An Intervention to Reduce Elderspeak." *Gerontologist* 43 (2): 242–247.

Williams, Kristine N. 2011. "Elderspeak in Institutional Care for Older Adults." In *Communication in Elderly Care: Cross-Cultural Perspectives*, edited by Peter Backhaus, 1–19. London: Bloomsbury.

———. 2013. "Evidence-Based Strategies for Communicating with Older Adults in Long-Term Care." *Journal of Clinical Outcomes Management* 20 (11): 507–512.

Williams, Kristine N., Ruth Herman, Byron Gajewski, and Kristel Wilson. 2009. "Elderspeak Communication: Impact on Dementia Care." *American Journal of Alzheimer's Disease and Other Dementias* 24 (1): 11–20.

Williams, Kristine N., Yelena Perkhounkova, Ruth Herman, and Ann Bossen. 2016. "A Communication Intervention to Reduce Resistiveness in Dementia Care: A Cluster Randomized Controlled Trial." *Gerontologist* 57 (4): 707–718.

Wills, T. A. 1991. "Social Support and Interpersonal Relationships." In *Prosocial Behavior*, edited by Margaret S. Clark, 265–289. Newbury Park, CA: Sage.

Windsor, Tim D., Rachel G. Curtis, and Mary A. Luszcz. 2015. "Sense of Purpose as a Psychological Resource for Aging Well." *Developmental Psychology* 51 (7): 975–986.

Yaden, David Bryce, Jonathan Iwry, and Andrew Newberg. 2016. "Neuroscience and Religion: Surveying the Field." In *Mental Religion*, edited by Niki Kasumi Clements, 277–299. New York: Macmillan.

Yafeh, Orit. 2007. "The Time in the Body: Cultural Construction of Femininity in Ultraorthodox Kindergartens for Girls." *Ethos* 35 (4): 516–553.

Index

Note: Page numbers in *italic type* refer to illustrative matter.

About the Author

ANNA I. CORWIN is a linguistic and psychological anthropologist. She received her PhD from the University of California–Los Angeles, and is an assistant professor of anthropology at Saint Mary's College of California. Her research and teaching interests span the fields of linguistic anthropology, psychological anthropology, the anthropology of religion, aging, and well-being. Corwin is a recipient of fellowships from the National Science Foundation and the National Endowment for the Humanities for her research on aging and well-being. Her work has been published in the *Journal of Linguistic Anthropology*; *HAU: Journal of Ethnographic Theory*; *Gender and Language*; *Medical Anthropology*; *Ethos*; and the *Gerontologist*.